Daoyin Yangsheng
Gong Shi Er Fa

other books in the same series

Da Wu
Health Qigong Da Wu Exercises
Chinese Health Qigong Association
ISBN 978 1 84819 192 1

Mawangdui Daoyin Shu
Qigong from the Mawangdui Silk Paintings
Chinese Health Qigong Association
ISBN 978 1 84819 193 8

Shi Er Duan Jin
12-Routine Sitting Exercises
Chinese Health Qigong Association
ISBN 978 1 84819 191 4

Taiji Yangsheng Zhang
Taiji Stick Qigong
Chinese Health Qigong Association
ISBN 978 1 84819 194 5

Ba Duan Jin
Eight-Section Qigong Exercises
Chinese Health Qigong Association
ISBN 978 1 78592 984 7

Yi Jin Jing
Tendon-Muscle Strengthening Qigong Exercises
Chinese Health Qigong Association
ISBN 978 1 78592 978 6

Daoyin Yangsheng Gong Shi Er Fa

12-Movement Health Qigong for All Ages

CHINESE HEALTH QIGONG ASSOCIATION

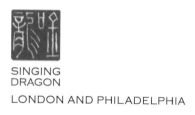

SINGING
DRAGON
LONDON AND PHILADELPHIA

The accompanying online materials can be downloaded at
www.jkp.com/voucher using the code
NAUJUBE

This edition published in 2014
by Singing Dragon
an imprint of Jessica Kingsley Publishers
73 Collier Street
London N1 9BE, UK
and
400 Market Street, Suite 400
Philadelphia, PA 19106, USA

www.singingdragon.com

First published by Foreign Languages Press, Beijing, China, 2012

Library of Congress Cataloging in Publication Data
A CIP catalog record for this book is available from the Library of Congress

British Library Cataloguing in Publication Data
A CIP catalogue record for this book is available from the British Library

ISBN 978 1 84819 417 5

Printed and bound by CPI Group (UK) Ltd, Croydon CR0 4YY

CONTENTS

The accompanying online materials can be downloaded at
www.jkp.com/voucher using the code
NAUJUBE

CHAPTER 1

Origins

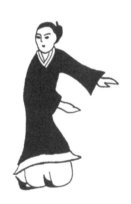

Chapter I
Origins

"*Daoyin*" was a kind of fitness exercise which combined breathing with limb movements in ancient China. The *Pictures of Daoyin Exercises* painted on a piece of silk from the Mawangdui Tombs of the Western Han Dynasty (206 BC–AD 25) unearthed in Changsha, Hunan Province in 1973 not only demonstrates fitness exercises and medical treatment such as "*yinlong*" (deafness prevention) and "*yinxiang*" (neck stretching), but also introduces limb movements and breathing exercises, such as "*yanghu*," similar to modern chest expansion. In addition, it contains exercises imitating animal movements, such as "*xiongjing*" (bear climbing a tree) and "*xin*" (bird stretching its legs).

Health preservation was developed and perfected in ancient China in order to enhance physical and mental health and proactively prevent illness after people gradually learnt about the relations between mankind and nature and the changes and the laws of physiological activities and the occurrence of illness. *Huangdi Neijing* (The Yellow Emperor's Cannon of Medicine),

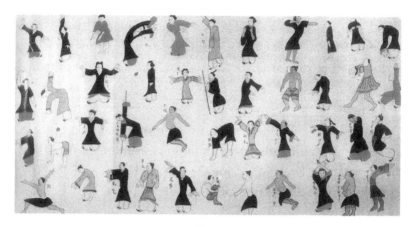

Fig. 1

an ancient Chinese medicinal bible, emphasizes the importance of illness prevention rather than its treatment. With this idea, the ancient people created a complete set of methods for health preservation, and some of them have developed into therapies for illness treatment.

The Chinese health preservation theory not only stresses the concept of "illness prevention prior to treatment," it also emphasizes good health and fitness. It is to fully stimulate the potential inner vitality of the body, advocate "temperance" and "harmony," and prevent various organs from injury.

As people acquainted themselves more with pathogenesis, they also put forward the theory of maintaining the spirit as well as the body in order to improve physical health and organ functions for illness prevention. The *Suwen* (Plain Questions) suggests that for the sake of physical health and vigorous energy people should abide by the laws of natural change, and institute health preservation strategies in line with these laws. In order to strengthen physical health, prolong life and prevent illness, people should form regular habits of eating and drinking, living, labor and rest. Irregular living and inordinate eating and drinking would impair the body's resistance to illness, affect physical health and bring about illness.

Meanwhile, in ancient times people paid special attention to the significant role of spirit cultivation in enhancing physical and mental health and preventing illness. All human beings are emotional, and emotions can alter their behavior and activities as well as the status of the viscera, even leading to physiological or pathological changes. Traditional Chinese Medicine (TCM) classifies seven emotions – happiness, anger, worry, yearning, sorrow, horror and surprise. Generally, these seven emotions, as people's mental responses to their peripheral environment, are normal physiological phenomena. However, excessive emotion and melancholy will bring about internal injury, impairing the five internal organs. Commonly, anger harms the liver, joy harms the heart, yearning harms the spleen, sorrow harms the lungs and horror harms the kidneys. Therefore, TCM suggests that the secret of physical and mental health lies in reducing malign spiritual stimulations and avoiding excessive emotional fluctuations; in other words, to keep a broad mind, smooth heart and optimistic attitude.

The 12-step *Daoyin* Health Preservation Exercises, compiled on the principle of health preservation in line with mental cultivation, forms a complete set of meridian exercises combining mental concentration, breath control and body movement for life vitality.

Mind

In ancient times people discovered that mental concentration could actively help to adjust the body and mind, keep a stable status inside the body, promote the balance of *yin* and *yang*, and lead to physical and mental health. This coincides with the concepts of "mind leading *qi*, *qi* leading blood and blood circulation dispelling illness" described by the ancient *qigong* and the *daoyin* theories.

However, in the course of mind cultivation, a "moderate degree" is especially stressed by the 12-step *Daoyin* Health Preservation Exercises. This is because the mind is regarded as being like water and fire: water can not only float a boat, but can also sink it; fire can bring warmth, but can also burn. Moderate mind concentration is the most important for practicing the 12-step *Daoyin* Health Preservation Exercises. If we don't concentrate the mind at all, the effect will be discounted, but if we concentrate the mind excessively it will cause deviations. Therefore, for mind concentration, the 12-step *Daoyin* Health Preservation Exercises need a "combination of mind and movement, just like a clear brook flowing calmly."

Qi

As early as more than 2,000 years ago, the Chinese people realized that *qi* is the mother of all life in Heaven and on Earth. Mankind is formed by the aggregation of *qi*, and so the 12-step *Daoyin* Health Preservation Exercises pays attention to breathing regulation on the basis of mind concentration and body movement. "Movement and breath should follow each other," which means reconciling and harmonizing delicate, constant, deep and long abdominal breathing with slow and gentle movements. The requirement of breathing regulation is to circulate the *qi* to the navel every time, inhaling and exhaling like an immortal turtle.

Form

Form refers to the corporeal body, including the viscera, skin and flesh, tendons and bones as well as meridians filled with vigor and blood. TCM suggests that "The form embodies the spirit which can't exist without it." This means that maintenance of the corporeal body (including maintenance of vigor) is crucial. In practicing the 12-step *Daoyin* Health Preservation Exercises, for instance, a skewed form may cause blockage of *qi*; blockage of *qi* may bring unease of spirit; unease of spirit may impair the effect of the practice.

We should notice that mind, *qi* and form are interactive and three-dimensional. The "mind practice" should follow "*qi* practice," because an easy spirit doesn't exist without fluent *qi*; "*qi* practice" can't be separated from "mind practice," because *qi* always follows the mind. However, mind and *qi* must be associated with "form practice," because form assists mind and *qi*, and a fluent *qi* and an easy spirit both come from proper form. That is to say that mind, *qi* and form are integrated as a whole. All of them play significant roles in physical fitness, health preservation and illness prevention. Therefore, they are regarded as the essences of the 12-step *Daoyin* Health Preservation Exercises.

CHAPTER II

Features and Effects

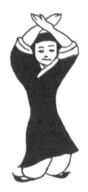

The 12-step *Daoyin* Health Preservation Exercises is a meridian fitness exercise which can promote the functions of the viscera and prevent illness, featuring easy-to-learn movements with abundant cultural connotations.

1. Principles and Methods of Health Preservation

The 12-step *Daoyin* Health Preservation Exercises actually originates from the theories of *I Ching* (*The Book of Changes*) and TCM health preservation.

Firstly, the 12-step *Daoyin* Health Preservation Exercises emphasizes the effect on life produced by movement, just as "running water is never stale and the door-hinge will never get worm-eaten," and lays stress on the health preservation concepts of "avoiding excessive movement and laboring in moderate degree." This is the embodiment of the two divinations of Heaven and Earth, dominating the *yang* movement and the *yin* stillness, respectively.

Secondly, each of the 12-step *Daoyin* Health Preservation Exercises is harmonious and symmetrical, embodying left and right, upper and lower, front and back and high and low motions. These harmonious and symmetrical motions are symbols of *"yin accompanying yang* making up the Way" and "closing following opening as Changes," as described in *The Book of Changes*, an application of the even reflections of the rise and fall as well as the changes of the *yin* and *yang* of the Eight Diagrams.

Thirdly, the 12-step *Daoyin* Health Preservation Exercises attaches importance to the cultivation of the essence, *qi* and spirit, and lays stress on "nourishing the spirit through regulating the mind," "practicing *qi* through regulating the breath" and "circulating meridians through regulating the form." It values the mutual rise and fall of the "kidney water" and "heart fire" in normal situations, and regards the interaction of the kidneys and the heart as an important link influencing the *yin-yang* balance throughout the body. It also stresses the avoidance of injury, with illness prevention prior to illness treatment. All this reflects the philosophy of *The Book of Changes* and TCM.

Fourthly, from the names of the movements we can see the profound influence of *The Book of Changes* and TCM on the exercises. Typical examples are the first and second movements – *"Qian Yuan Qi Yun"* (Beginning of Heaven's Creation) and *"Shuang Yu Xuan Ge"* (Double Fish Hung on the Wall) (see details from the meanings of the names of movements).

Fifthly, the 12-step *Daoyin* Health Preservation Exercises requires the practitioner to face the light to practice according to the idea of the rise and fall and conversion between *yin* and *yang* in *The Book of Changes*.

Sixthly, it requires certain timing for exercise which embodies the changing law of the rise and fall between *yin* and *yang* as described in *The Book of Changes* and by TCM. It is the best to do exercises outdoors at dawn, inhaling and exhaling, and doing *daoyin* (other time periods are also recommended), because dawn is the time when the *yang qi* is produced in the human body and in nature, and it helps the circulation of meridian, *qi* and blood.

2. Circular Movement and Integration of Man and Nature

All things and creatures in the universe from the Galaxy and the Solar System in the macrocosm to cells, atoms, electrons and protons are constantly circulating, connecting and developing in a circular way.

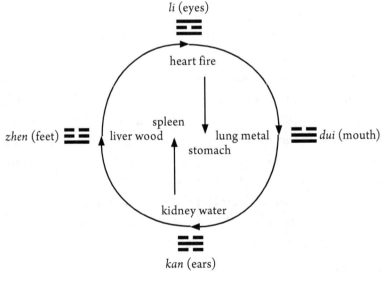

Fig. 2

The rising and falling movements of the human viscera also follow a circular movement with spleen and stomach in the middle, the heart above, kidneys below, liver left and lungs right.

The circulation of the *qi* and blood along the 12 meridians of the human body is also in the form of a circle (Table 1).

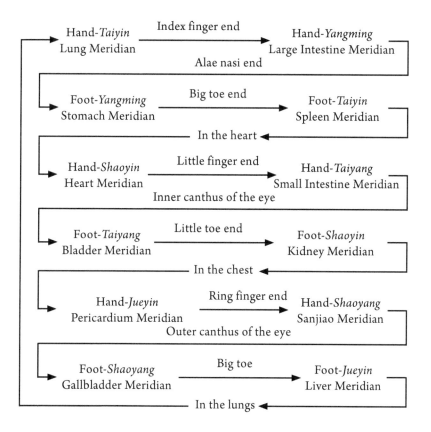

Table 1 The circulation along the 12 meridians

In the 12-step *Daoyin* Health Preservation Exercises, each movement is executed in circles of different sizes, including hand, foot and body movements, in continuous, cycled, repeated modes like silkworms making silk, clouds drifting and water flowing.

The circles of different sizes exactly correspond to the circular paths of the different parts of the human body and the circular paths of all the things in the universe. They not only increase the flexibility of all the joints of the body, but also strengthen the muscles, bones and ligaments. Even more important is its reflection of the coordination between the rise and fall of the movements and the *qi* circulation of the internal organs, and the harmonious relationships between man and nature, which means the "harmony of man with nature." This undoubtedly has certain effects on improving the physique, preventing and treating illnesses, and prolonging life.

3. Rotating in Movements, with Effects on Tips

The 12-step *Daoyin* Health Preservation Exercises is composed of 12 sets of movements, stressing "rotating during movement," "movement starting from rotation", and "posture stopping during rotation." This has the following advantages:

1) It can increase stimulus to the nerves, bones, muscles and joints to improve the functions of the nervous system, harden the bones, develop and strengthen the muscles, and improve the flexibility and stability of the joints.

2) As the muscles and ligaments have a bigger drawing force on the bones because of the rotating movements, the latter help

to improve the quality of the red marrow of the hematopoietic system.

3) It can increase the stimulus to the meridian channels and acupoints on the whole body, and help to smooth the channels, promote the flow of *qi* and blood, remove food stagnation and dispel blood stasis.

While stressing rotation during movement, the Exercises attach special importance to the "effect on the tips." The tips refer to wrists, ankle joints, fingers and toes, the remote parts of the limbs. TCM believes that the source acupoints of the three hand *yin* meridians, three hand *yang* meridians, three foot *yin* meridians and three foot *yang* meridians are near the joints of the wrists and ankles.

The source acupoints are the parts of the internal organs where the original *qi* flows through or ends. The pathological change of a certain organ is often shown at the source acupoint. The source acupoints play an important role in preventing and treating diseases of the internal organs. They are: lungs – *taiyuan*, large intestine – *hegu*, stomach – *chongyang*, spleen – *taibai*, heart – *shenmen*, small intestine – *wangu*, bladder – *jinggu*, kidneys – *taixi*, xinbao – *daling*, triple energizers – *yangchi*, gallbladder – *qiuxu*, and liver – *taichong*.

During the exercises, the regular physical activities of the wrist and ankle joints are, in fact, auto-massage of the above 12 source acupoints. They can improve the *qi* and blood flow through the channels, harmonize the physiological functions of *yin* and *yang*, improve the pathological immune function and the reflection of symptoms through the meridians, and strengthen the preventive and treatment functions of conducting the response of the meridians and adjusting emptiness and solidity to produce the effect of maintaining the genuine *qi* (energy), relieving the internal organs and improving the physique and health.

Moreover, rhythmic movements of the fingers and toes help to start and stimulate the normal functioning of the meridian channels in the whole body for the smooth flow of *qi* and blood to achieve the effect of "no pain when the channels are thorough," and help to maintain the balance of *yin* and *yang* of the organism for the purpose of strengthening the body and prolonging life. Snapping the fingernails, stretching the palms, clenching the fists, forming hooked hands, turning the toes up and toes grasping the ground in the exercises are the movements designed for this purpose.

4. Concentrating Mind with Correct Movements

Mind refers to will and thought, and movement refers to posture. When doing the exercises movements with correct postures are required; this is *daoyin* by movement. Distracting thoughts should be dismissed, and the mind concentrated; this is *daoyin* by mind. Moreover, it also requires the close combination of *daoyin* by mind and *daoyin* by movement. The purpose for the combination is to achieve the effect of strengthening the body and preserving health, although the movements vary and the acupoints for mind concentration are different.

Daoyin by mind is in fact a process in which the psychological activities of man influence his physiological activities. It is "seeking movement in stillness." In other words, use "stillness" to stimulate the blood circulation in the whole body, improve the *qi* function of the internal organs, smooth the flow of *qi* and blood in the meridians, and open the orifices of the acupoints.

5. Breathing Follows Movement and Slow Movement Goes with Long Breathing

In performing the Health Preservation Exercise, breathing should follows movement, and slow movement goes with long breathing. Soft and slow movements are keys to breathing exercise. This is to seek stillness in movement so as to promote the regulation of *qi* and blood in the meridians, the balance between *yin* and *yang* of the internal organs, the soothing of the *qi* functions of the heart and lungs, and the tranquility of the nervous system.

"Breathing" in the 12-step *Daoyin* Health Preservation Exercises refers to soft, even, deep and long abdominal respiration, and a breath includes inhaling and exhaling. As the movements in the exercise are soft and slow, the breathing must be soft, even, deep and long. Only in this way can it be ensured that breathing follows movement.

How to ensure the coordination of movement and breathing? In the exercises, inhale first and then exhale, inhale while rising and exhale while dropping, inhale while opening and exhale while closing, inhale through nose and exhale through nose or mouth.

6. Strengthening the Inside While Assisting the Outside, Concentrating on the Waist

"Strengthening the inside while assisting the outside, concentrating on the waist" is another important characteristic of the 12-step *Daoyin* Health Preservation Exercises. It means that the exercises aim first to improve the functions of the internal organs of the human body, thereby improving the functions of the limbs, skeleton, tendons, blood vessels, muscles, skin and bones.

TCM holds that the liver, heart, spleen, lungs and kidneys are the five *zang* organs, and belong to *yin*, and the gallbladder, small intestine, large intestine, stomach, bladder and triple energizers are the six *fu* organs, and belong to *yang*. The five *zang* organs manage the stored essence of life, while the six *fu* organs manage the growth of things. *Yang* manages the outside, while *yin* manages the inside. *Zang* and *fu*, *yin* and *yang*, outside and inside, cooperate with each other to guarantee good health for the human body.

Therefore, the improvement of the functions of the five *zang* organs and the six *fu* organs is the foundation for keeping the limbs, skeleton, tendons, blood vessels, muscles, skin, bones, five sense organs and nine body orifices in good health. This is the main reason why the exercises put great emphasis on "strengthening the inside and assisting the outside."

Life hinges on the waist. This refers to the activities of the lumbar area as the key point for the exercise, because the lumbar vertebra is the primary joint of the human body for bending, flexion and extension. TCM holds that an important point in the lumbar area is located at the *mingmen* acupoint in the depression below the spinous process of the second lumbar vertebra. Physicians believe that the *mingmen* acupoint is the major acupoint for long life. If the *mingmen* is exhausted, the life ends. Moreover, there is also another important acupoint on the *Ren* meridian, that is, the *shenque* acupoint, as *daoyin* specialists call it – the major acupoint for long life. *Shenque* is the center of the navel, which faces the *mingmen* acupoint on the *Du* meridian. When people do the fourth, fifth and sixth steps of the Exercises with the waist as the axis, the *Du* meridian, the kidneys at the lumbar area and *mingmen* acupoint, and the *Ren* meridian, and the spleen and stomach, through the *zhongjiao* and *shenque* acupoints, are stimulated, resulting in communication between the front and rear parts of the body, and the integration of *yin* and *yang*, thus producing the effect of prolonging life to a certain degree. At the same time, the *Du* meridian travels along the inside of the spinal column and joins the collateral in the brain. The brain is an extremely important organ in the human body. When the brain is full, a man is strong and can do heavy work; when the brain is empty, a man is weak, and feels dizzy, with ringing in the ears, aching at the waist, dim-sighted, lethargic and tired.

This is the main reason why the 12-step *Daoyin* Health Preservation Exercises regards "life hinges on the waist" as the principle of "*daoyin* for health perservation."

Movements

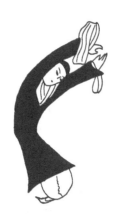

Section I Names of the Movements

Initial Stance

Step 1 Beginning of Heaven's Creation (*Qian Yuan Qi Yun*)

Step 2 Double Fish Hung on the Wall (*Shuang Yu Xuan Ge*)

Step 3 Old Horse Stabled (*Lao Ji Fu Li*)

Step 4 Ji Chang Shoots a Louse (*Ji Chang Guan Shi*)

Step 5 Bending the Body to Brush the Shoes (*Gong Shen Dan Xue*)

Step 6 Rhinoceros Gazes at the Moon (*Xi Niu Wang Yue*)

Step 7 Lotus Flower Appears Above the Water (*Fu Rong Chu Shui*)

Step 8 Golden Rooster Heralds the Dawn (*Jin Ji Bao Xiao*)

Step 9 Wild Geese Land on the Beach (*Ping Sha Luo Yan*)

Step 10 White Crane Flies High in the Clouds (*Yun Duan Bai He*)

Step 11 Phoenix Salutes the People (*Feng Huang Lai Yi*)

Step 12 *Qi* and Breath Return to the Origin (*Qi Xi Gui Yuan*)

Ending Stance

Section II Movements (Standing Stance)

Initial Stance

1. Guide to the movements

Stand erect with the feet together, and relax the whole body (Fig. 3).

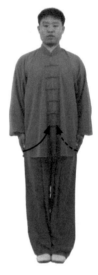

Fig. 3

2. Essential points

1) Close the eyes slightly and look straight forward, tip of the tongue touching the hard palate, and clench the teeth.

2) Read the following rhyme silently while doing the exercise:

Ye lan ren jing wan lv pao

Yi shou dan tian feng qi qiao

Hu xi xu huan da que qiao

Shen qing ru yan piao yun xiao

(Dispel all thoughts in the deep night,

Concentrate the mind on the *dantian* with closed orifices.

Breathe slowly to build a magpie bridge,

Let the body fly like a swallow in the clouds.)

3. *Points for attention*

1) Put the hands on the *dantian* (lower belly), with the right hand over the left (Fig. 4).

2) After finishing reciting the rhyme, put the hands down by the sides, eyes looking straight ahead (Fig. 5).

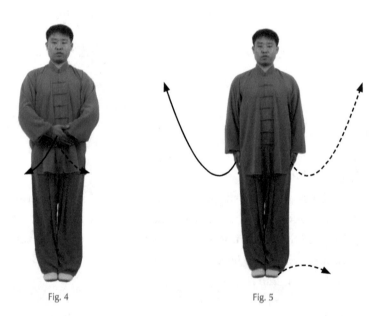

Fig. 4   Fig. 5

Step 1 Beginning of Heaven's Creation (*Qian Yuan Qi Yun*)

1. Meaning of the name

The Book of Changes says: "乾 (qian), 元 (yuan), 亨 (heng), 利 (li), 贞 (zhen)." The four characters "元 (yuan), 亨 (heng), 利 (li), 贞 (zhen)" are the commentaries on various combinations of the Eight Trigrams for the character 乾 (qian).

乾 (qian) is the beginning of all the phenomena of nature and all things on the earth. It is also said that all phenomena of nature and all things on the earth were created by the functions of 乾 (qian), and therefore it was called "元 (yuan)." "亨 (heng)" refers to 亨通 (heng tong). It means there is no obstruction. "利 (li)" also means smooth passage. "贞 (zhen)" means backbone or pillar. This is the meaning of "乾元启运"(beginning of Heaven's creation), and it is used to dispel the interferences of distracting thoughts or worries in the practitioner's mind.

2. Guide to the movements

1) While breathing in, raise the anus and pull in the abdomen. Shift the body weight onto the right foot, slightly bend the right leg, and move the left foot to the left, so that the feet are slightly wider than shoulder-width apart. The toes point forward. As the body weight is shifted to between the feet, straighten the legs. At the same time, swing the palms to the right and left, respectively, and to shoulder level as the arms are rotated inward, palms facing backward, and arms naturally straight, eyes fixed on the left palm (Fig. 6). As the arms are turned outward, swing the palms level to

in front of the body, palms facing down and shoulder-width apart, arms naturally straight, eyes fixed on both palms (Fig. 7).

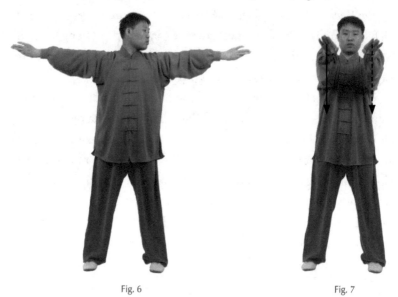

Fig. 6   Fig. 7

2) While breathing out, relax the abdomen and anus, and bend the legs to squat down. At the same time, move the palms with the arms slightly back and drop them down to the level of the navel, palms facing down and fingertips pointing forward, eyes looking straight ahead (Fig. 8).

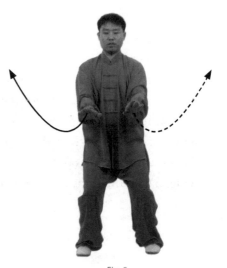

Fig. 8

3) While breathing in, raise the anus, pull in the abdomen, and straighten the legs slowly. At the same time, rotate the palms inward with the elbows and swing them respectively to the left and right to shoulder level, palms facing backward, arms naturally straight, eyes fixed on the right palm (Fig. 9). Without stopping, shift the body weight onto the right foot, right leg half bent and left leg naturally straight. At the same time, rotate the palms outward with the arms and swing them in front of the body level, palms facing down and shoulder-width apart, and arms naturally straight, eyes fixed on both palms (Fig. 10).

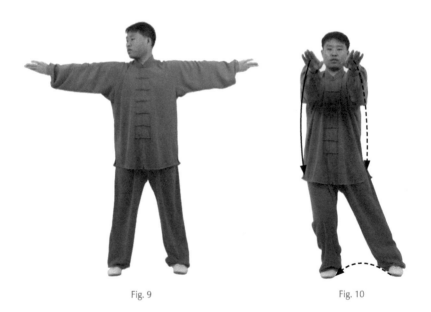

Fig. 9   Fig. 10

4) While breathing out, relax the abdomen and anus, move the left foot next to the right foot, and straighten the bent legs slowly. At the same time, press the palms downward to navel level and drop them by the sides. Stand with the feet together, eyes looking straight ahead (Fig. 11).

Do Movements 5, 6, 7 and 8 the same as Movements 1, 2, 3 and 4, but in the opposite direction.

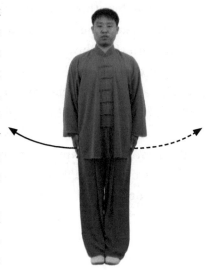

Fig. 11

3. Number of times to practice
Do one round.

4. Points for attention
1) Exert slight force to the thumbs to increase the range of rotation of the arms when rotating the arms inward and moving the palms apart.

2) The degree of the squatting action differs from person to person.

3) Make the sound "*hu*" silently or concentrate the mind on the *dantian*.

5. Main effects

1) It helps to smooth the hand-*taiyin* lung meridian and the hand-*yangming* large intestine meridian, and has a certain effect in preventing and treating diseases of the respiratory system, such as colds and bronchitis.

2) Concentrating the mind on the *dantian* helps to expel distracting thoughts, purify the cerebrum, invigorate the spleen, replenish *qi*, strengthen the body's resistance, consolidate the constitution and improve the physique.

3) The formula for respiration says: The exhaling sound of "*hu*" is attached to the spleen. Therefore, make the sound "*hu*" silently to regulate the stomach function and invigorate the spleen.

Step 2 Double Fish Hung on the Wall (*Shuang Yu Xuan Ge*)

1. Meaning of the name

"Double Fish Hung on the Wall" originally refers to two fish of different colors with the head and tail connected, representing *yin* and *yang*, hung on a wall. It denotes the growth and decline of *yin* and *yang* and the transformation between them in nature.

In this case, they refer to the movement: Keep the feet together, press one hand downward to the side of the hips while holding the other hand forward above the head.

2. Guide to the movements

1) While breathing in, raise the anus, pull in the abdomen, and straighten the legs. At the same time, rotate the palms with the arms inward, and swing them respectively to the left and right sides, arms straight and slightly below shoulder level, palms facing backward, eyes looking straight to the left (Fig. 12). While breathing out, relax the abdomen and anus, turn the body to the right, shift the body weight onto the right foot, right leg half bent, left heel up to form a left T-stance. At the same time, rotate the left palm with the left arm outward, and move it back to in front of the right lower abdomen, palm facing up. Then move the right palm inward, and drop it down onto the left wrist, with the phalanx of the ring finger placed on the *taiyuan* acupoint as if feeling the pulse, eyes fixed on the hands (Fig. 13).

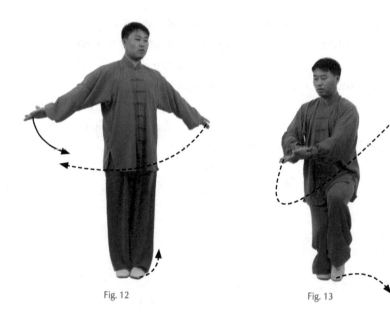

Fig. 12   Fig. 13

2) While breathing in, raise the anus, pull in the abdomen, turn the body to the left, and move the left foot forward to the left to change the empty stance into a bow stance. At the same time, keep the hands in the same posture of feeling the pulse, and swing them forward in a curved line to the left in front of the body, left arm naturally straight and left palm facing up, eyes fixed on both palms (Fig. 14). While breathing out, shift the body weight back, turn the body to the right to form a left empty stance, left toes turned up. At the same time, rotate the left arm inward and the right arm outward. After twisting the finger on the *taiyuan* acupoint, put the right palm on the left in front of the chest, palm to palm and *laogong* acupoint to *laogong* acupoint, palms about 20 cm apart from the chest, eyes fixed on both palms (Fig. 15).

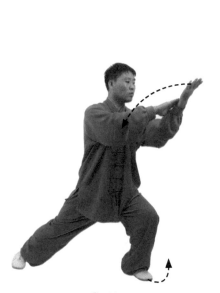

Fig. 14

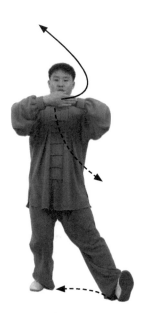

Fig. 15

3) While breathing in, raise the anus, pull in the abdomen, move the left foot to the right to keep the feet together, and straighten the bent legs gradually. At the same time, rub the palms to and fro horizontally, and then rotate the left palm with the left arm inward to press downward to the side of the left hip, about 20 cm from the hip, left arm bent into an arc, left fingers facing right, and rotate the right palm with the right arm inward to raise the arm above the head to the right, right arm bent in an arc, right fingers facing left, eyes looking straight to the left (Fig. 16).

4) While breathing out, relax the abdomen and anus. At the same time, keep the left hand in the same position, and press the right palm slightly down and forward with the right arm and

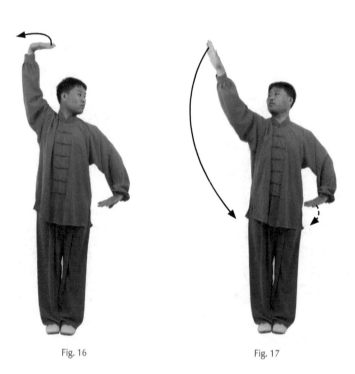

Fig. 16   Fig. 17

elbow dropped to the right, eyes turning to the right palm (Fig. 17). Without stopping, move the right palm down, put both palms by the sides, and stand with the feet together, eyes looking straight ahead (Fig. 18).

Do Movements 5, 6, 7 and 8 the same as Movements 1, 2, 3 and 4, but in the opposite direction.

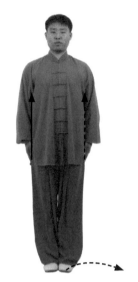

Fig. 18

3. Number of times to practice

Do one round.

4. Points for attention

1) Breathe in and breathe out once each for the first and second movements, and keep the breath deep, long and slow.

2) Rotate the body with the waist as the axis in the second movement to bring along the palms.

3) When feeling the pulse, place the ring finger, middle finger and index finger at the end of the palm.

4) There should be no stagnation in breathing. The movements are continuous, and the upper and lower limbs are fully coordinated.

5) Make the sound "*hu*" silently or concentrate the mind on the *dantian* (refer to the *guanyuan* acupoint).

5. Main effects

1) Helps to improve the function of the lungs and relieve disorders of the respiratory system such as cough and asthma.

2) Helps to improve the functions of the spleen and stomach, and relieve disorders of the digestive system such as indigestion and stomachache.

3) Improves the function of the kidneys, and has a certain effect on the reproductive and the urinary systems.

Step 3 Old Horse Stabled (*Lao Ji Fu Li*)

1. Meaning of the name

"Old Horse Stabled" is a quote from Cao Cao (a military strategist, statesman and writer during the Three Kingdoms period): "An old steed in the stable still aspires to gallop a thousand *li*, an old man of high endeavor cherishes great ambition." These movements evoke people of endeavor who still have ambitions although they are old.

2. Guide to the movements

1) While breathing in, raise the anus, pull in the abdomen, shift the body weight onto the right foot, right leg slightly bent, and move the left foot apart to the left (about the length of three feet of the practitioner), and straighten the legs gradually as the body weight is shifted to between the feet. At the same time, rotate the palms with the arms outward and swing them forward to shoulder level, palms facing up and shoulder-width apart, eyes fixed on both palms (Fig. 19). While breathing out, relax the abdomen and anus. At the same time, clench the fists gradually, and move them with

the arms, elbows bent, back in front of the chest, elbows facing down, forearms touching each other against the body, fists as high as the chin, and eyes looking straight ahead (Fig. 20).

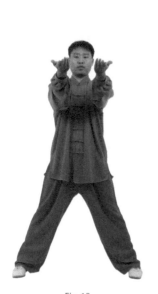

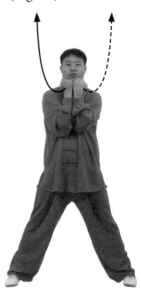

Fig. 19   Fig. 20

2) While breathing in, raise the anus, pull in the abdomen, unclench the fists into palms, rotate them inward and extend them forward above, palms facing forward and arms naturally straight, palms shoulder-width apart, eyes looking straight ahead (Fig. 21). While breathing out, relax the abdomen and anus, and bend the legs to form a horse-riding stance. At the same time, hook the wrists gradually (connecting the *shaoshang* and *shangyang* acupoints), and move them from the sides to hang behind the body, with the points of the hooks facing up, arms straight, eyes looking straight to the left (Fig. 22).

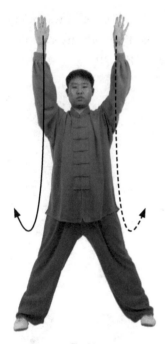

Fig. 21

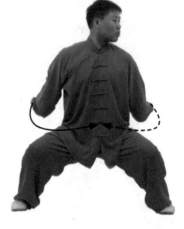

Fig. 22

3) While breathing in, raise the anus and pull in the abdomen, without moving the legs. At the same time, straighten the hooked hands and rotate them inward with the arms before the abdomen, the backs of the hands facing each other, fingers facing down, eyes looking straight ahead (Fig. 23). Without stopping, straighten the legs. At the same time, bend the wrists and hands, and press back the first, second and third fingers one by one in order. Move them apart, and let them hang by the right and left sides of the body, arms naturally straight, fingers facing up, wrists as high as shoulder level, eyes looking straight ahead (Figs. 24–26).

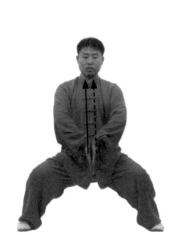

Fig. 23

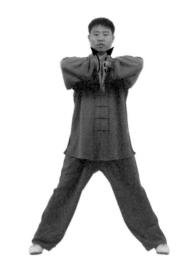

Fig. 24

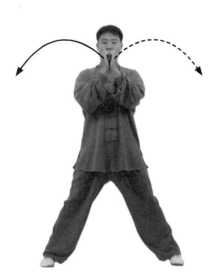

Fig. 25

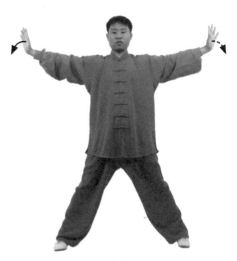

Fig. 26

4) While breathing out, relax the abdomen and anus, shift the body weight onto the right foot, right leg half-bent, move the left foot beside the right foot, and straighten the legs slowly. At the same time, drop the palms lightly from the sides down to form a standing stance, eyes looking straight ahead (Figs. 27 and 28).

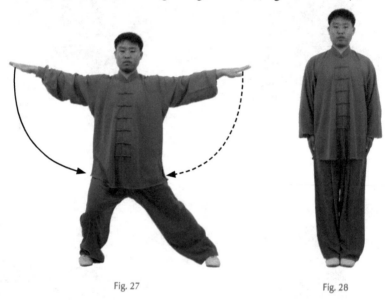

Fig. 27   Fig. 28

Do Movements 5, 6, 7 and 8 the same as Movements 1, 2, 3 and 4, but in the opposite direction.

3. Number of times to practice
Do one round. Clench the fists at the eighth movement, and place them by the waist in preparation for Step 4 (Fig. 29).

4. Points for attention
1) It is appropriate to breathe in and breathe out once each at the first and second movements, and keep the breath deep, long and slow.

2) When clenching the fists with bent elbows in front of the chest, use the middle fingertip to touch the *laogong* acupoint.

3) The height of the horse-riding stance varies from person to person, but the wrists must be bent fully for the hooked hands.

4) Make the sound "*dzer*" silently, concentrate to direct the movements or concentrate the mind on the *taiyuan* acupoint.

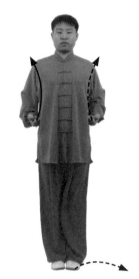

Fig. 29

5. Main effects

1) Pressing the *laogong* acupoint helps to improve the function of the heart and has a certain effect of relieving high blood pressure and combating coronary heart disease.

2) Hooking the hands, hooking the wrists and doubling the fingers help to invigorate the heart and lungs as they have the effect of massaging *taiyuan*, the source acupoint of the lung meridian, *daling*, the source acupoint of the pericardium meridian, and *shenmen*, the source acupoint of the heart meridian.

3) Helps to supplement the spleen *qi* and increase the primordial *qi* to strengthen the body's resistance and improve the health.

4) Uttering silently the sound "*dzer*" helps to invigorate the lungs.

Step 4 Ji Chang Shoots a Louse (*Ji Chang Guan Shi*)

I. Meaning of the name

"Ji Chang Shoots a Louse" is the title of a story relating how Ji Chang apprenticed himself to the expert archer Fei Wei in ancient times. The master told him: "If you want to learn to shoot arrows well, you must see a very small object as a very large one, and see a vague object very clearly." So Ji Chang went home, caught a louse, and hung it up tied to the tail hair of an ox. He faced south and fixed his eyes on the louse every day. Three years later, the louse looked as big as a cart wheel to him, while other things looked like as big as hills. He made a bow and shot an arrow straight through the louse, leaving the ox tail hair intact.

2. Guide to the movements

1) While breathing in, raise the anus, pull in the abdomen, shift the body weight onto the right foot, right leg half bent, move the left leg a big step to the left, toes facing forward, and straighten both legs immediately. At the same time, push the palms held vertically forward, arms naturally straight, wrists about shoulder level, palms shoulder-width apart and fingers up, eyes fixed on both palms (Fig. 30).

2) While breathing out, relax the abdomen and anus, turn the body to the left, bend the left leg and keep the right leg straight. The heels should press the ground. At the same time, clench the fists at first loosely, and move them horizontally to behind the body as it is turned to the left, relax the left arm at shoulder level, bend the right arm, with the right elbow in front of the left chest, eyes fixed on the left fist (Fig. 31). Without stopping, continue to turn the body slightly to the left, clench the fists tightly, fingers touching the *laogong* acupoint. Straighten the left arm and extend

the left fist sideways. Pull the right fist back to in front of the right side of the chest, drop the hips and relax the chest, eyes fixed on the left fist (Figs. 32-1 and 32-2).

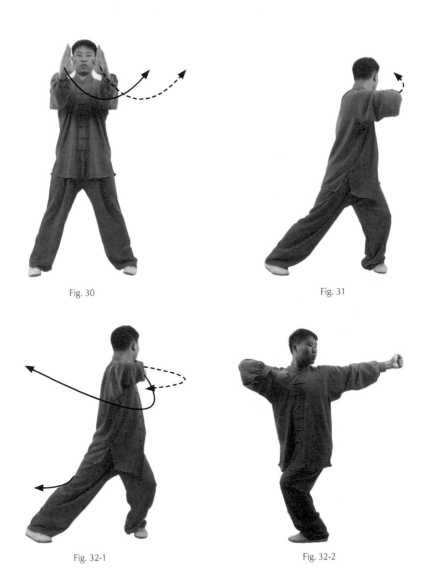

Fig. 30

Fig. 31

Fig. 32-1

Fig. 32-2

3) While breathing in, raise the anus, pull in the abdomen, turn the body to the right to keep it upright, rotate the right heel inward, toes forward, and then shift the body weight onto the right foot, with the right leg bent. At the same time, unclench the fists and move them horizontally to in front of the body as the arms are rotated inward, arms straight at should level, palms facing down, eyes fixed on both palms (Fig. 33).

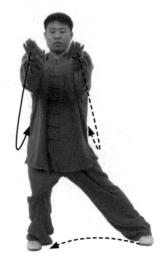

Fig. 33

4) While breathing out, relax the abdomen and anus, move the left foot to put the feet together, and straighten the legs gradually. At the same time, turn the palms down, clench the fists and move them back by the sides of the waist, palms, facing up, and eyes looking straight ahead (Fig. 34).

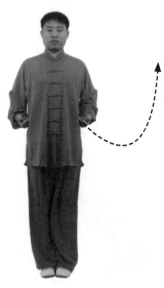

Fig. 34

Do Movements 5, 6, 7 and 8 the same as Movements 1, 2, 3 and 4, but in the opposite direction.

3. Number of times to practice

Do two rounds.

4. Points for attention

1) When pushing the palms forward in the first movement, it is appropriate for the force to originate at the root (shoulders), flow through the middle (elbows) and reach the tips (hands).

2) When turning the body to the left in the second movement, it is appropriate to keep the upper part of the body upright, and make sure that the heels do not leave the ground.

3) When doing the third movement, it is appropriate to lower the body weight, and first look at the left palm and then look at both palms when the body is upright again.

4) When doing the fourth movement, raise the *baihui* acupoint, drop the shoulders and elbows with the hands down, and send *qi* to the *dantian*.

5) Concentrate the mind on the *mingmen* acupoint.

5. Main effects

1) Clenching the fists and touching the *laogong* acupoint helps to clear the heart of heat and reduce temperature.

2) "Pulling the bow and shooting the arrow" helps to relax the chest and promote the normal flow of *qi*, and regulate the heart and lungs.

3) Concentrating the mind on the *mingmen* acupoint and pressing the heels to the ground sideways to twist the *yongquan*

acupoint helps to nourish *yin* and the kidneys, and strengthen the kidneys and the waist.

Step 5 Bending the Body to Brush the Shoes
(*Gong Shen Dan Xue*)

1. Meaning of the name

Bending the body means bending the body forward as if bowing. Brushing means removing dust. "Bending the body to brush the shoes" means removing dust and harmful matter from the surface of the human body on the one hand, and on the other, it means dispelling all distracting thoughts, evil thoughts in particular, from the mind to purify the brain, relieve mental strain and strengthen the body.

2. Guide to the movements

1) While breathing in, raise the anus, pull in the abdomen, relax the chest, stretch the body to its fullest extent, and turn the body to the left. At the same time, clench the left fist and extend it up with the left arm rotated inward, eyes fixed on the left palm (Fig. 35).

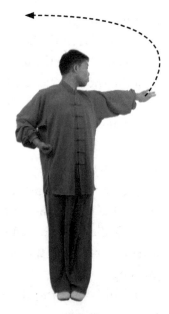

Fig. 35

Without stopping, swing the left palm forward above to the right with the left arm rotated outward and the body turned to the right, straighten the left arm, eyes fixed on the left palm (Fig. 36). Without stopping, drop the left palm to in front of the right shoulder (the back of the thumb and the radial side of the index finger against the right shoulder), bend the left elbow and turn up the fingers, eyes fixed on the left palm (Fig. 37).

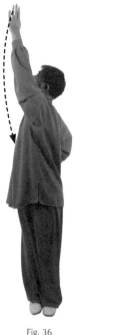

Fig. 36

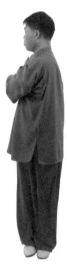

Fig. 37

2) While breathing out, relax the abdomen and anus, bend the upper body to the right side, legs straight. At the same time, use the left palm to rub the right leg downward with the left arm rotated outward (the phalanxes along the foot-*taiyang* bladder meridian, the palm along the foot-*shaoyang* gallbladder meridian and the palm base along the foot-*yangming* stomach meridian, reaching the outer ankle), head raised slightly (Fig. 38). Without stopping, turn the body to the left to keep it upright. At the same time, the left palm, as the left arm is rotated inward, rubs the left leg from the instep to the outer ankle of the left foot as if brushing the shoes, head raised slightly, eyes fixed on the left palm (Fig. 39).

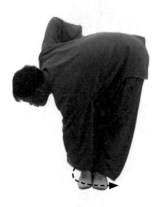

Fig. 38

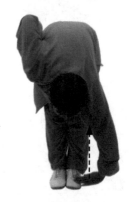

Fig. 39

3) While breathing in, raise the anus and pull in the abdomen. At the same time, clench the left fist as the left arm is rotated outward, and raise it to the left knee joint as the upper body rises a bit, head slightly raised (Fig. 40).

4) While breathing out, relax the abdomen and anus, and straighten the upper body. At the same time, move the left fist back to the side of the waist, the bent fingers facing up, the *zhongchong* acupoint at the tip of the middle finger touching the *laogong* acupoint at the center of the palm, eyes looking straight ahead (Fig. 41).

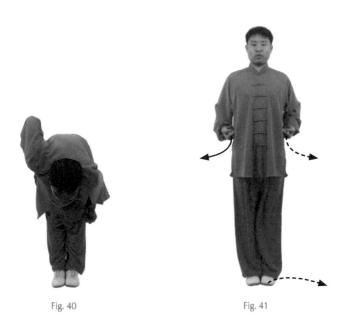

Fig. 40   Fig. 41

Do Movements 5, 6, 7 and 8 the same as Movements 1, 2, 3 and 4, but in the opposite direction.

3. Number of times to practice
Do two rounds.

4. Points for attention
1) Concentrate the mind on the *mingmen* acupoint.
2) Relax the body as much as possible, and make a large range of movement. Straighten the legs when "bending forward to brush the shoes." Beginners and people with ailments should choose a range of movement within their ability.
3) The body should be straightened slowly and evenly.
4) People suffering from high blood pressure should raise the head when practicing this step.

5. Main effects
Bending the body forward can act on the waist and the *Du* meridian which runs through the spinal column and connects with the kidneys. The waist is the location of the essence of the kidneys. According to *yin* and *yang* theory, the kidneys and the bladder connect with each other, and the bladder meridian passes through the waist. Moreover, the *Du, Chong* and *Dai* meridians are also located in the waist. Therefore, regular practice of the movement of "bending the body to brush the shoes" helps to nourish the *yin* of the kidneys, warm and nourish the *yang* of the bladder, take in *qi* and return it to the kidneys, invigorate the kidneys and loins, and invigorate the brain.

Step 6 Rhinoceros Gazes at the Moon (*Xi Niu Wang Yue*)

1. Meaning of the name

An ancient Chinese tradition holds that the horn of the rhinoceros has white, thread-like lines, which connect the tip of the horn to the animal's brain. So a rhinoceros' horn is called a "sensitive horn." "Rhinoceros gazes at the moon" describes the movement of turning the body to improve the functions of the loins and kidneys in particular.

2. Guide to the movements

1) While breathing in, raise the anus, pull in the abdomen, shift the body weight onto the right foot, right leg bent, and move the left foot a big step to the left, toes facing forward. At the same time, unclench the fists, and press the palms down and backward as the arms are rotated inward, eyes looking straight ahead (Fig. 42).

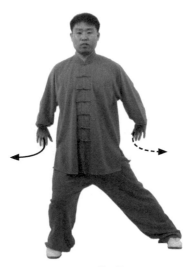

Fig. 42

Without stopping, shift the body weight onto the left foot, left leg bent and right leg straight. At the same time, continue to rotate the arms inward, relax the bent palms and swing them upward in a curved line to the two sides slightly behind the back, eyes looking straight ahead (Fig. 43).

2) While breathing out, relax the abdomen and anus, use the front sole of the right foot as the axis, press the heels on the ground and facing outward, turn the upper body to the left, right leg straight and left leg bent. At the same time, swing both palms upward from the two sides and stop them above the forehead, both arms bent into curves, palms facing up and forward, fingers pointing to each other, eyes looking up and to the left as if watching the moon (Fig. 44).

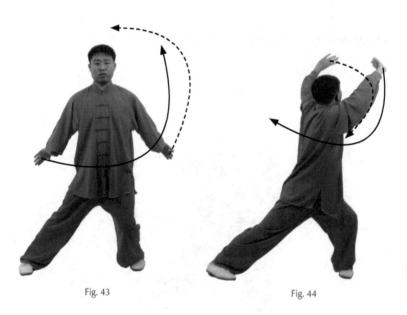

Fig. 43   Fig. 44

3) While breathing in, raise the anus, pull in the abdomen, and turn the body to the right to keep it upright. With the front sole of the right foot as the axis, rotate the heel inward to shift the body weight onto the right foot, right leg half bent and left leg straight, toe pointing forward. At the same time, move the palms downward and swing them in a curved line to before the chest as the arms are rotated outward, arms naturally straight, palms facing up and fingers forward, palms shoulder-width apart, eyes fixed on both palms (Fig. 45).

4) While breathing out, relax the abdomen and anus, move the left foot to the right to put the feet together again, and straighten the legs gradually. At the same time, after dropping the palms and putting them by the sides of the body as the arms are rotated inward, continue to clench the fists, and move them back to the sides of the waist, palms facing up, eyes looking straight ahead (Fig.46).

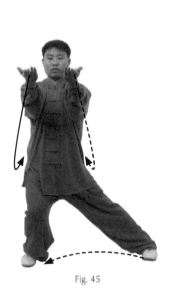

Fig. 45

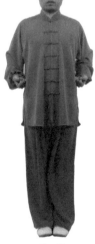

Fig. 46

Do Movements 5, 6, 7 and 8 the same as Movements 1, 2, 3 and 4, but in the opposite direction.

3. Number of times to practice

Do two rounds, drop the palms by the sides of the body and stand with feet together at the eighth movement of the second round, eyes looking straight ahead (Fig. 47).

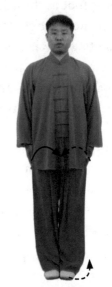

Fig. 47

4. Points for attention

1) Concentrate the mind on the *mingmen* acupoint.

2) It is appropriate to turn the waist with a big range of movement, lower the hips, kneel down with the left knee or right knee (depending on the starting direction), and straighten the rear leg with the right heel on the ground.

3) When clenching the fists, the *zhongchong* acupoint should touch the *laogong* acupoint for an instant.

4) It is appropriate to rotate the arms with a big range of movement at an even speed. Be sure not to stiffen the shoulders and avoid rotating the arms at an uneven speed.

5. Main effects

1) By turning the neck and rotating the waist, this step helps to relax the muscles of the neck, back and waist, and relieve pain in the shoulders, elbows, wrists, neck, back and waist.

2) By removing the obstacles from the three *yin* meridians and three *yang* meridians of the hands, it helps to strengthen the heart, improve the functions of the lungs, clear and regulate the *Sanjiao* meridian, moisten the intestines, and resolve the nodes.

3) By concentrating the mind on the *mingmen* acupoint and pressing the heel on the ground sideways to twist the *yongquan* acupoint, it helps to nourish *yin* and the kidneys.

Step 7 Lotus Flower Appears Above the Water
(*Fu Rong Chu Shui*)
1. Meaning of the name

In Step 7, the cross-legged sitting stance looks like the twisted roots of the lotus flower. It likes water, but is not contaminated by mud. The body rises up, with the bases of the palms against each other held up like a lotus flower blooming.

2. Guide to the movements

1) While breathing in, raise the anus, pull in the abdomen, shift the body weight onto the right foot, right leg slightly bent, left heel up. At the same time, keep the backs of the hands against each other in front of the abdomen, fingers facing down, eyes looking straight ahead (Fig. 48). Without stopping, move the left foot to the left, slightly wider than shoulder-width, shift the body weight immediately to between the feet, both legs straight. At the same time, flex the carpuses, the metacarpal bones, the first phalanxes, the

second phalanxes and the third
phalanxes of the hands one after
another in order and proceed to
snap the fingernails to unclench
the fists, and move them apart
to the two sides, palms raised
to shoulder level, and arms
naturally straight, palms facing
up, eyes looking straight ahead
(Figs. 49 and 50).

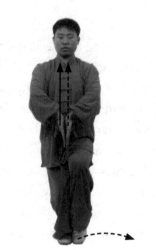

Fig. 48

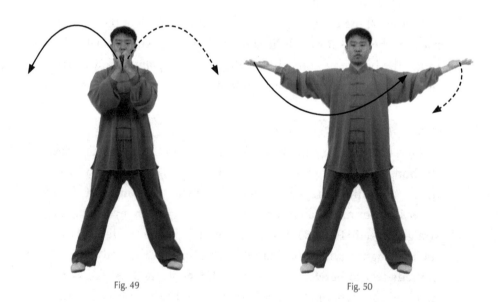

Fig. 49   Fig. 50

2) While breathing out, relax the abdomen and anus, shift the body weight onto the left foot and turn the body to the left. At the same time, clench the left fist as the left arm is rotated inward, elbow bent, and drop the fist slightly, clenched fingers facing down; clench the right fist as the right arm is rotated inward, and swing it forward horizontally to the left, the clenched fingers facing down, eyes fixed on the right fist (Fig. 51). Without stopping, move the right foot backward to the left behind the left foot and squat down into a cross-legged sitting stance. At the same time, drop the left fist down to the left hip, left arm bent into a curve, wrist up, fist top facing backward, fist about 30 cm from the hip; move the right fist back to in front of the right side of the chest, with the body turned to the right and the right arm rotated inward, wrist up and clenched fingers facing forward, fist about 30 cm apart from the chest, eyes looking straight ahead (Fig. 52).

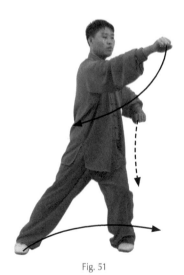

Fig. 51

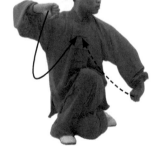

Fig. 52

3) While breathing in, raise the anus, pull in the abdomen, unclench the fists, move the right arm downward and the left arm upward, the bases of the palms against each other in front of the chest in the posture of a blooming lotus flower, eyes fixed on both palms (Fig. 53). Without stopping, move the right foot to the right to return to the original position, and straighten both legs gradually. At the same time, continue to hold the palms upward and extend the arms naturally, eyes fixed on both palms (Fig. 54).

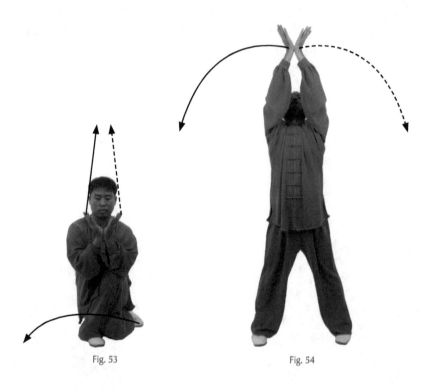

Fig. 53   Fig. 54

4) While breathing out, relax the abdomen and anus, shift the body weight onto the right foot, right leg slightly bent, move the left foot to put the feet together again, and straighten the bent legs. At the same time, drop the palms down by the sides of the body, eyes looking straight ahead (Figs. 55 and 56).

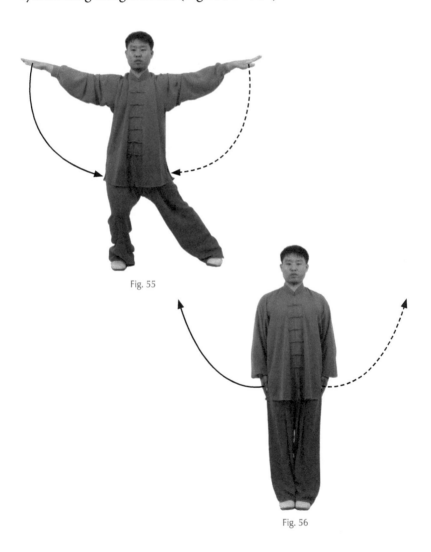

Fig. 55

Fig. 56

Do Movements 5, 6, 7 and 8 the same as Movements 1, 2, 3 and 4, but in the opposite direction.

3. Number of times to practice

Do one round.

4. Points for attention

1) When doubling the fingers and snapping the fingernails at the first movement, the movements of the shoulders, elbows, wrists and fingers should be continuous. Do the movement in a relaxed and elegant manner.

2) When bending the legs to squat down in a cross-legged sitting stance at the second movement, one arm is bent at the hip and the other is moved back to in front of the chest. The movements above and below must be uniform, with equal attention given to the hands and feet. The position should look like a lotus root in the mud and the lotus flower above the water.

3) When the body rises up at the third movement, hold up the palms, their bases against each other, in the symbolic posture of a lotus flower appearing above the water in a clear pond and in a soothing breeze.

4) At the fourth movement, move the left foot back together with the right, raise the *baihui* acupoint on the top of the head, drop the shoulders, straighten the neck, and drop the elbows, with hands hanging down by the sides.

5) Utter the sound "*si*" silently or concentrate the mind on the *taiyuan* acupoint.

5. Main effects

1) Removing obstacles from the three *yin* and three *yang* meridians of the hands helps to strengthen the heart, nourish the lungs, moisten the intestines, and regulate the *Sanjiao* meridian.

2) Removal of obstacles from the three *yin* and three *yang* meridians of the foot helps to regulate the stomach, invigorate the spleen, soothe the liver, promote the function of the gallbladder, and strengthen the kidneys and the waist.

3) This is an all-round exercise, and therefore helps to improve the functions of all internal organs.

Step 8 Golden Rooster Heralds the Dawn (*Jin Ji Bao Xiao*)

1. Meaning of the name

In this step, the practitioner stands on one leg and extends the other leg backwards. At the same time, the hands are joined to form a hook with the wrists raised above the head as if a rooster is crowing at dawn. Hence the name.

2. Guide to the movements

1) While breathing in, raise the anus, pull in the abdomen, raise the *baihui* acupoint on the top of the head, and straighten the legs, heels up. At the same time, change the hands gradually into hooks, and swing them upward to the two sides, arms naturally straight, and wrists about at shoulder level, eyes fixed on the left hooked hand (Figs. 57-1 and 57-2).

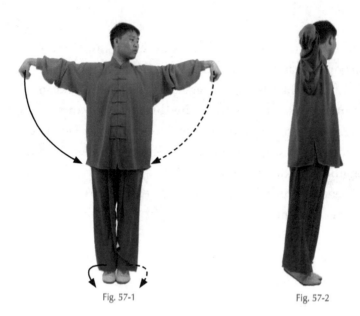

Fig. 57-1   Fig. 57-2

2) While breathing out, relax the abdomen and anus, heels down on the ground, and bend the legs, knees against each other. At the same time, change the hooked hands into flat palms, and press them down by the sides with the elbows slightly curved, arms naturally straight, palms facing down, and fingers outward, eyes looking straight ahead (Fig. 58).

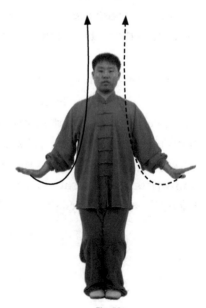

Fig. 58

3) While breathing in, raise the anus, pull in the abdomen, straighten the right leg, bend the left leg and extend it backwards, instep flattened and sole facing up. At the same time, while rotating the arms inward and moving the palms in a curved way inward before the abdomen, change the palms into hooked hands, extend the arms forward and upward to both sides of the head and above it, tips of the hooked fingers facing down, and arch the back, eyes looking straight ahead (Figs. 59-1 and 59-2).

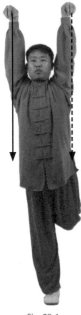
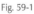
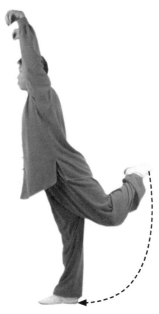

Fig. 59-1   Fig. 59-2

4) While breathing out, relax the abdomen and anus, drop the left foot downwards to beside the right foot to put feet together again, legs half bent. At the same time, change the hooked hands into flat palms and press them down by the hips, palms facing down and fingers facing forward, eyes looking straight ahead (Fig. 60).

Do Movements 5, 6, 7 and 8 the same as Movements 1, 2, 3 and 4, but in the opposite direction.

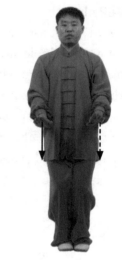

Fig. 60

3. Number of times to practice

Do one round. After finishing the last movement, straighten the legs gradually, and at the same time keep the feet together in a standing stance with the palms down by the sides, eyes looking straight ahead (Fig. 61).

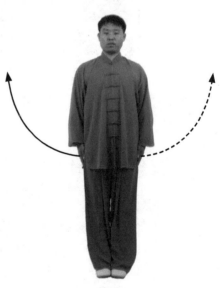

Fig. 61

4. Points for attention

1) Concentrate the mind on the *dantian* (referring to the *guanyuan* acupoint here)

2) Keep the upper and lower limbs coordinated, relaxed, soft, natural and elegant.

3) While standing on one leg, the toes of the supporting leg firmly against the ground, raise the *baihui* acupoint, eyes looking into the distance.

4) While swinging the hooked wrists and extending them upward, it's better to relax the chest and unfold the body, fully and naturally.

5) While breathing out, utter the sound "*chui*" softly.

5. Main effects

1) Pulling the heels up to press the *yongquan* acupoint helps to activate and start the kidney meridian of foot-*shaoyin* to nourish *yin* and the kidneys.

2) Forming hooked hands, swing them upward and changing them into flat palms before pressing them downwards helps to remove the obstacles from the source acupoints of the three *yin* and three *yang* meridians of the hand, to remove obstruction in the meridians and collaterals, nourish the heart and lungs, and regulate the *Sanjiao* meridian.

3) Uttering the sound "*chui*" nourishes *yin* and the kidneys.

Step 9 Wild Geese Land on the Beach (*Ping Sha Luo Yan*)

1. Meaning of the name

"Wild Geese Land on the Beach" is a musical piece for the *qin*, a traditional Chinese seven-stringed instrument. It is first recorded in the *Orthodox Ancient Qin* (1643). It describes the flying, landing and crying of wild geese on a beach. In this step, the movements of "squatting down with crossed-legs in a sitting position and pushing the palms with the wrists bent backwards" look just like geese on a beach. Hence the name.

2. Guide to the movements

1) While breathing in, raise the anus, pull in the abdomen, relax and unfold the body. At the same time, swing the palms with the top ends of the wrist joints leading to both sides of the body in curved lines to shoulder level, arms naturally straight, palms facing down, eyes fixed on the right palm (Fig. 62).

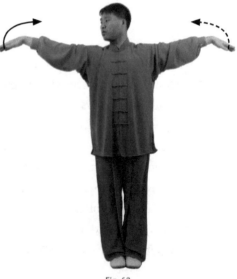

Fig. 62

Without stopping, shift the body weight onto the right foot, move the left foot backwards to the right behind the right foot. At the same time, move the palms downwards with the arms, elbows bent, and draw them back in an arc posture, palms as high as shoulder level and facing down, eyes fixed on the right palm (Fig. 63).

2) While breathing out, relax the abdomen and anus, bend the legs to squat down to a cross-legged sitting stance. At the same time, move the arms with the elbows straight and palms sitting on the wrists, and push them in curved lines to the sides, both arms naturally straight, wrists at shoulder level, palms facing outward and fingers facing up, eyes fixed on the right palm (Fig. 64).

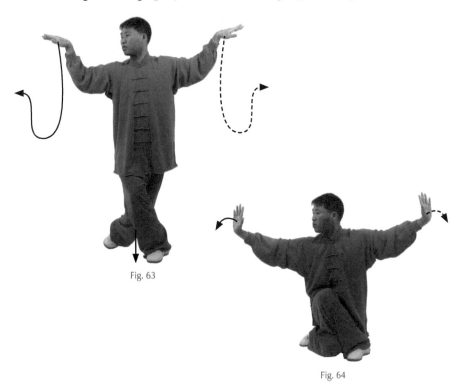

Fig. 63

Fig. 64

3) While breathing in, raise the anus, pull in the abdomen, move the legs upward slightly, relax the chest and unfold the body (keep the left foot behind the right foot). At the same time, extend the palms to the two sides, arms naturally straight, and palms facing down. Then, move the palms downwards, with the arms and elbows bent, and draw them back in an arc posture, palms as high as shoulder level and facing down, eyes fixed on the right palm (Fig. 65).

4) While breathing out, relax the abdomen and anus, bend the legs to squat down to a cross-legged sitting stance. At the same time, move the arms with the elbows straight and palms sitting on the wrists and push them in curved lines to the sides, both arms naturally straight, wrists at shoulder level, palms facing outward and fingers facing up, eyes fixed on the right palm (Fig. 66).

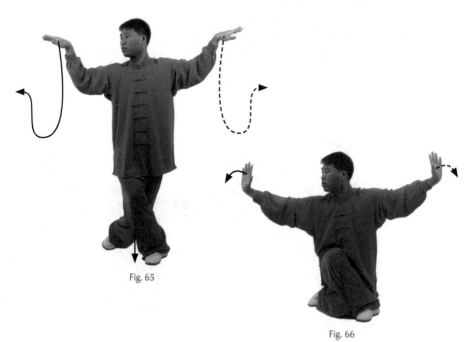

Fig. 65

Fig. 66

5) While breathing in, raise the anus, pull in the abdomen, and move the legs upward slightly, left heel still up. At the same time, extend the hands upward slightly to the sides and swing them to shoulder level, arms naturally straight, and palms facing down, eyes fixed on the right palm (Fig. 67).

6) While breathing out, relax the abdomen and anus, move the left foot to the right foot to keep them together, and straighten the bent legs. At the same time, keep the feet together in a standing stance with the palms down by the sides, eyes looking straight ahead (Fig. 68). Alternate the movements.

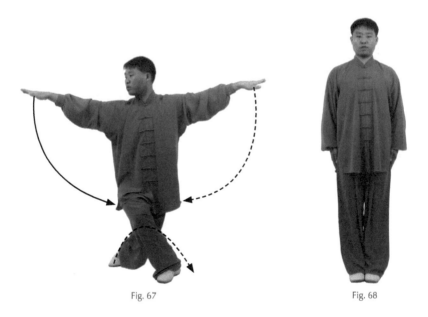

Fig. 67   Fig. 68

3. Number of times to practice

Do one round in each direction.

4. Points for attention

1) Concentrate the mind on the *laogong* acupoint.

2) Breathe in when raising and breathe out when lowering the body, relax the whole body, and keep the inner sides of the legs against each other in the cross-legged sitting stance.

3) Old and weak people or sufferers from chronic diseases may reduce the degree of difficulty, and change the cross-legged sitting stance to the resting stance.

4) When breathing out, utter the sound "*her*" softly.

5. Main effects

1) Concentrating the mind on the *laogong* acupoint helps to regulate the hand-*jueyin* pericardium meridian, relieve the heart and regulate the flow of blood.

2) Bending the legs to form the cross-legged sitting stance helps to remove obstruction from the meridians of the three *yin* and three *yang* of the foot, and improves the functions of the spleen, stomach, liver, gallbladder and kidneys.

3) Uttering the sound "*her*" helps to relieve the heart.

Step 10 White Crane Flies High in the Clouds
(*Yun Duan Bai He*)

1. Meaning of the name

People in ancient times often regarded white cranes as able and virtuous persons of moral integrity. In this step, the charm of the free, light, elegant and slow movement of "moving the hands upward to snap the wrists and flash the palms above the head" is just like that of a white crane flying in the sky. Hence the name.

2. Guide to the movements

1) While breathing in, raise the anus, pull in the abdomen, and straighten the legs, toes pointed up. At the same time, move the *hegu* acupoints on the palms as the arms are rotated inward to rub the sides of the body upward to near the *dabao* acupoint on the lateral side of the chest, eyes looking straight ahead (Fig. 69). Without stopping, rotate the palms with the *hegu* acupoints as the axes while the arms are rotated outward, so that the fingers face backward, eyes looking straight ahead (Fig. 70).

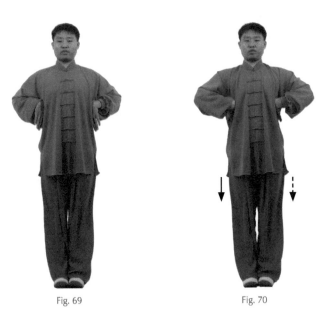

Fig. 69   Fig. 70

2) While breathing out, relax the abdomen and anus, and bend the legs slightly, toes grasping the ground. At the same time, press the backs of the hands to the *dabao* acupoints, and then put the backs of the hands together in front of the chest, both arms bent, and fingers facing inward, eyes looking straight ahead (Fig. 71). Without stopping, continue to bend the legs and squat down. At the same time, press the wrists against each other, bend the fingers and swing them respectively to the left and the right, arms naturally straight and at shoulder level, and palms facing forward, eyes looking straight ahead (Fig. 72).

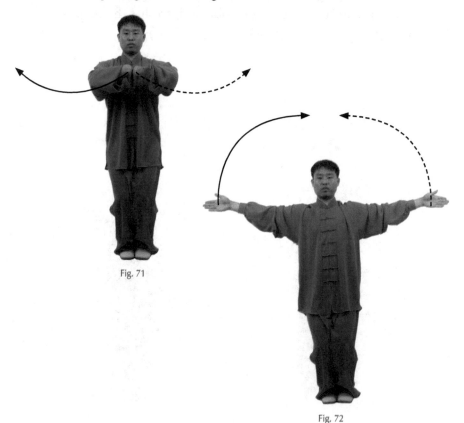

Fig. 71

Fig. 72

3) While breathing in, raise the anus, pull in the abdomen, and straighten the legs, heels up. At the same time, swing the palms up and forward above the head to the two sides as the arms are rotated inward, to snap the wrists and flash the palms, both arms bent in an arc, eyes looking straight ahead (Fig. 73).

4) While breathing out, relax the abdomen and anus, heels on the ground. At the same time, drop the palms downwards from the two sides, and stand with the feet together, palms down by the sides, eyes looking straight ahead (Fig. 74).

Do Movements 5, 6, 7 and 8 the same as Movements 1, 2, 3 and 4.

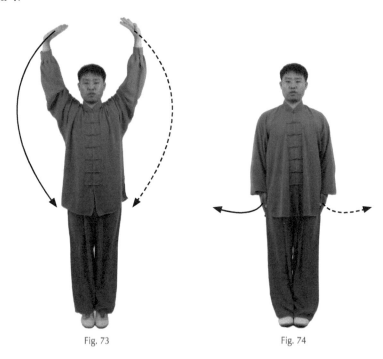

Fig. 73   Fig. 74

3. Number of times to practice
   Do one round.

4. Points for attention
   1) When keeping the heels fully up and rubbing the *dabao* acupoint with the *hegu* acupoint at the first movement, it's appropriate to relax the chest, straighten the back, and raise the *baihui* acupoint on the top of the head.
   2) When doing the second movement, bend the legs to squat down, and keep the inner sides of the legs against each other. When swinging the palms respectively to the left and right, it's better to start with the wrists against each other, and bend the fingers one by one in order, and move them continuously.
   3) At the third movement, raise the *baihui* acupoint on the top of the head to pull the whole body upward. When snapping the wrists and flashing the palms, keep the ends of the middle fingers and the *jianyu* acupoint on the shoulders basically at the same level.
   4) At the fourth movement, drop the shoulders and elbows together with the hands, *qi* flowing to the *dantian*.
   5) Concentrate the mind on the *dantian* (referring to the *guanyuan* acupoint here).

5. Main effects
   1) Pulling up the toes to press the *yongquan* acupoint of the foot-*shaoyin* kidney meridian activates the meridians, and nourishes *yin* and the kidneys.
   2) Using the *hegu* acupoint to twist the *dabao* acupoint helps to moisten the intestines, resolve the nodes, regulate the stomach and invigorate the spleen.

3) Snapping the wrists and flashing the palms overhead helps to regulate the *Sanjiao* meridian and remove obstacles from the *shuidao* acupoint at the lower abdomen.

Step 11 Phoenix Salutes the People (*Feng Huang Lai Yi*)
1. Meaning of the name

The phoenix, a legendary auspicious bird, was one of the "four spirits" of ancient Chinese mythology. The unicorn, turtle and dragon were the others. The phoenix was also regarded as the king of birds. "The phoenix saluting the people" was an auspicious sign.

2. Guide to the movements

1) While breathing in, raise the anus, pull in the abdomen, straighten the legs and turn the body 45 degrees to the left. At the same time, rotate the palms with the arms first inward and then outward, and swing them from the sides to shoulder level, arms naturally straight, palms shoulder-width apart and facing up, eyes looking straight to the left (Figs. 75 and 76).

2) While breathing out, relax the abdomen and anus, shift the body weight onto the right foot, right leg half bent, and move the left foot forward to the left to form an empty stance. Immediately afterwards, shift the body weight onto the left foot, right heel up, and both legs straight. At the same time, rotate the palms with the arms inward and gradually hook the hands (*shaoshang* and *shangyang* acupoints connected) and stretch them behind the body, arms straight and hook tips facing up, eyes looking straight ahead to the left (Figs. 77 and 78).

Movements

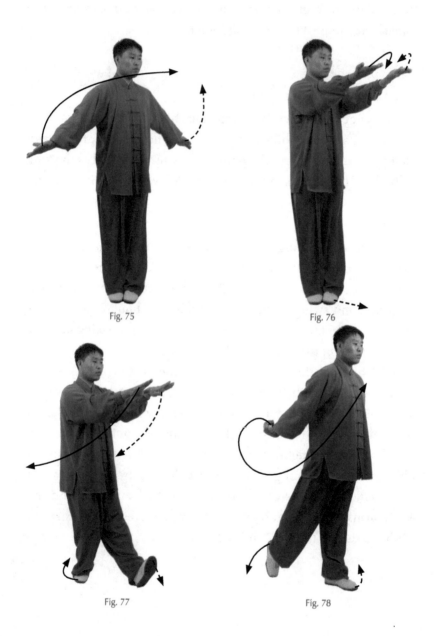

Fig. 75

Fig. 76

Fig. 77

Fig. 78

3) While breathing in, raise the anus, pull in the abdomen, shift the body weight backward, toes of the front foot turned up, and turn the body back and keep it upright. At the same time, change the hooked hands into palms, move them from the sides of the waist and cross them in front of the chest, left palm inside and facing the inside, eyes fixed on both palms (Fig. 79). Without stopping, rotate the palms with the arms, move them before the face and apart to the two sides, arms naturally straight, wrists at shoulder level, and fingers facing up, eyes looking straight ahead (Fig. 80).

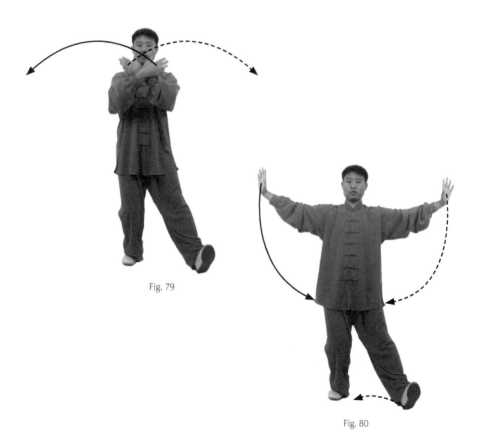

Fig. 79

Fig. 80

4) While breathing out, relax the abdomen and anus, move the left foot to the right foot to keep them together, and straighten the bent legs. At the same time, drop the palms downward on the two sides, and stand with the feet together, palms down by the sides, eyes looking straight ahead (Fig. 81).

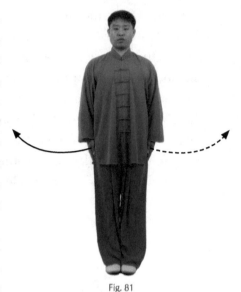

Fig. 81

Do Movements 5, 6, 7 and 8 the same as Movements 1, 2, 3 and 4, but in the opposite direction.

3. Number of times to practice

Do one round.

4. Points for attention

1) At the first movement, raise the *baihui* acupoint at the top of the head, keep the body upright and turn the spinal column to drive the arms apart and make them swing forward.

2) At the second movement, change the empty stance from bent leg to straight leg; the movement of raising the heel of the rear foot should reflect the characteristics of continuity and roundness. The time for bending the wrists of the hooked hands should be short and the movement slightly forceful.

3) At the third movement, when moving the hands and palms apart in front of the chest and turning the face to the left and right, keep the chest relaxed and the back straight, relax the waist and keep the hips tucked in.

4) At the fourth movement, move the left foot to the right foot to keep them together. Raise the *baihui* acupoint at the top of the head to straighten the whole body.

5) Concentrate the mind on the *dantian*, and utter the sound "*hu*" softly.

5. Main effects

1) Turning the body and rotating the arms helps to remove obstruction from the *Ren* and *Du* meridians and the three *yin* meridians and three *yang* meridians of the hand.

2) Bending the wrists to form hooked hands stimulates the well points and source acupoints of the three *yin* and three *yang* meridians of the foot, and therefore helps to improve the functions of the heart, lungs, large intestine and small intestine.

3) Turning up the toes stimulates the source acupoints of the three *yin* and three *yang* meridians of the foot, and therefore helps to improve the functions of the liver, gallbladder, spleen, stomach, bladder and kidneys.

4) Uttering the sound "*hu*" soothes and relieves the stomach and spleen.

Step 12 Qi and Breath Return to the Origin (*Qi Xi Gui Yuan*)

1. Meaning of the name

For this step, the practitioner should attach importance to the collection of *yang qi*, but also to the collection of *yin qi*. As ancient health preservation specialists said, for the purpose of preserving health, people should also pay attention to receiving *yin qi* from the earth apart from absorbing *yang qi* from the sun and Heaven. When practicing the 12-step *Daoyin* Health Preservation Exercises, one should accept equal amounts of *yin qi* and *yang qi*, depending on one's specific conditions. This is because it is extremely easy to consume *yin*, and so *yin qi* is often insufficient while *yang qi* is often more than enough. Therefore, *qigong* and *daoyin* specialists believe that the best time for doing exercises is dawn and early morning, because this is the best time for the generation of *yang qi* in the human body and the natural environment, and the time which manifests the biggest density of the "negative ions" good for the physiological functions of all systems of the human body.

2. Guide to the movements

1) While breathing in, raise the anus and pull in the abdomen. At the same time, rotate the palms with the arms first inward and then outward, and swing them to the two sides of the body, palms changing from facing backward to facing forward. The angle between the arms and the upper body should be about 60 degrees, arms naturally straight, eyes looking straight ahead (Figs. 82 and 83).

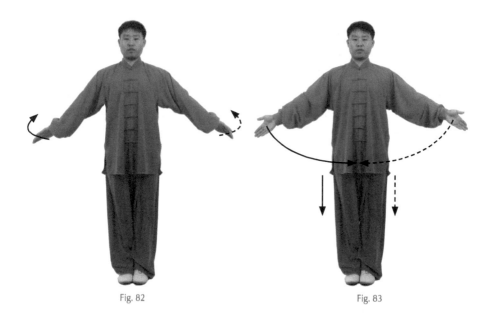

Fig. 82

Fig. 83

2) While breathing out, relax the abdomen and anus, and bend the legs. At the same time, move the palms back inward to form a circle before the lower abdomen, fingers pointing to each other, and return the *qi* of essence from the sun and the moon to the *guanyuan* acupoint, eyes looking straight ahead (Fig. 84).

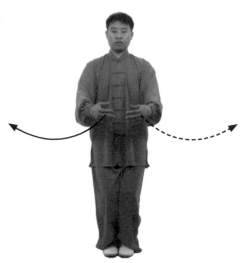

Fig. 84

3) While breathing in, raise the anus, pull in the abdomen and straighten the legs. At the same time, rotate the palms with the arms first inward and then outward, and swing them to the two sides of the body, palms changing from facing backward to facing forward. The angle between the arms and the upper body should be about 60 degrees, arms naturally straight, eyes looking straight ahead (Figs. 85 and 86).

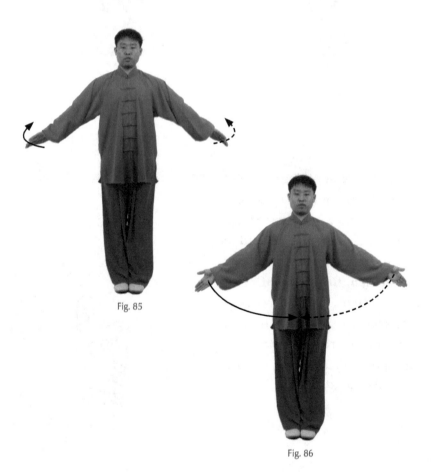

Fig. 85

Fig. 86

4) The same as Movement 2.

5) The same as Movement 3.

6) While breathing out, relax the abdomen and anus, and keep the legs naturally straight. At the same time, move the palms back inward to put one over the other at the *guanyuan* acupoint, left hand inside for the male and right hand inside for the female, eyes looking straight ahead (Fig. 87).

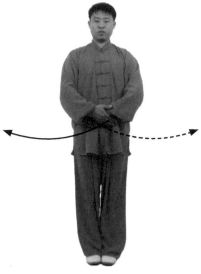

Fig. 87

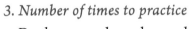

3. *Number of times to practice*

Do three rounds, each round including breathing in once and breathing out once.

4. *Points for attention*

1) Concentrate the mind on the collection of *qi* for the *guanyuan* acupoint.

2) When breathing in, raise the *baihui* acupoint at the top of the head, and when breathing out, relax the waist, keep the hips in and the body upright, and relax the whole body.

3) When moving the palms back inward to collect *qi* of essence from the sun and the moon, pay attention to narrowing the passage for the flow of *qi* so as to accelerate it.

5. Main effects

The *guanyuan* acupoint is located on the *Ren* meridian, and is one of the acupoints of the *dantian*. It is the meeting point for the three *yin* meridians of the foot and the *Ren* meridian and one of the front *mu* points of the small intestine meridian. TCM calls it the "major acupoint of long life," and it has a noticeable effect in preserving health. Therefore, using the mind to draw in *qi* for the *guanyuan* acupoint helps to invigorate the central *qi*, nourish the origin *qi*, nourish the internal organs and regulate *yin* and *yang*.

Ending Stance

1. Guide to the movements

1) While breathing in, raise the anus, and pull in the abdomen. At the same time, rotate the palms with the arms first inward and then outward, and swing them to the two sides. Change the direction of the palms from facing backward to facing forward. The angle between the arms and the upper body should be about 60 degrees, arms naturally straight, eyes looking straight ahead (Figs. 88 and 89).

2) While breathing out, relax the abdomen and anus, and straighten the legs naturally. At the same time, move the palms back inward to put one over the other at the *guanyuan* acupoint, left hand inside for the male and right hand inside for the female, eyes lightly closed (Fig. 90).

3) Execute the movement of the "red dragon (tongue) stirs the sea," three times each to the left and right parts of the mouth so as to increase the elixir (saliva) and swallow it in three gulps.

4) After finishing the movements, put the palms down by the sides, and end the step slowly to finish the whole set of exercises (Fig. 91).

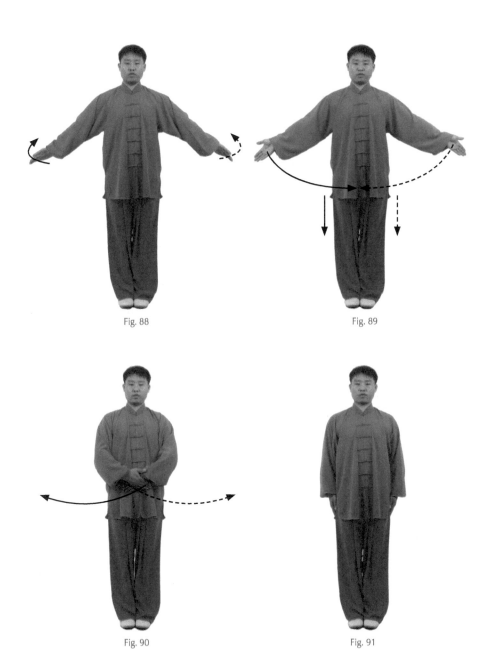

Fig. 88

Fig. 89

Fig. 90

Fig. 91

2. Points for attention

    1) Concentrate the mind on the elixir (saliva).

    2) Swallow the elixir with a clear sound.

3. Main effects

    1) Huangfu Long, a centenarian in the period of the Three Kingdoms (220–280), said: "People should drink jade water every morning to be strong and in good health... Jade water is the saliva in the mouth... After rinsing the mouth in the morning, the mouth is full of saliva. Just swallow it. This is called refining the essence" (from *Prescriptions Worth a Thousand Pieces of Gold for Emergencies*).

    2) Cheng Guopeng, a famous physician of the Qing Dynasty (1644–1911), says in his *Medical Science* that saliva is "the best prescription for treating deficiency of *yin.*"

    3) Modern medical research demonstrates that saliva contains globulin, mucous protein, amino acid, amylose, lysozyme, immuneglobulin, and trace elements.

    4) The Chinese character "活" (live, living) is a combination of "氵 or 水" and "舌," meaning the water by the side of the tongue. In this case, water just means saliva.

    5) A Japanese scholar says after research that saliva is the natural agent for the prevention of cancer, and has the function of making carcinogenic substances harmless.

    6) Modern research demonstrates that saliva helps to improve glycometabolism, and has the effect of keeping the blood sugar constant.

Section III Movements (Sitting Stance)

Initial Stance

1. Guide to the movements

Sit in a chair with the body upright, feet shoulder-width apart, toes pointing forward, the *laogong* acupoints on the palms touching the *futu* acupoint on the anterior side of the upper thigh, head erect and neck straight, chin slightly tucked in, and eyes looking straight ahead or lightly closed (Figs. 92 and 93)

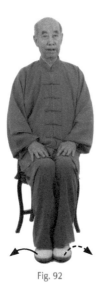

Fig. 92

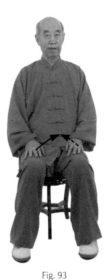

Fig. 93

2. Essential points

1) Close the lips lightly, tongue touching the palate, and upper and lower teeth touching.

2) Read the following rhyme silently while doing the exercises:

Ye lan ren jing wan lv pao
Yi shou dan tian feng qi qiao
Hu xi xu huan da que qiao
Shen qing ru yan piao yun xiao
 (Dispel all thoughts in the deep night,
  Concentrate the mind on the *dantian* with closed orifices.
  Breathe slowly to build a magpie bridge,
  Let the body fly like a swallow in the clouds.)

3. Points for attention

1) Place the hands one on top of the other at the *dantian* (lower belly), with the right hand over the left (Fig. 94).

2) After reciting the rhymes, drop the hands down to the *futu* acupoint. Keep the body upright, neck straight and head erect, eyes looking straight ahead (Fig. 95).

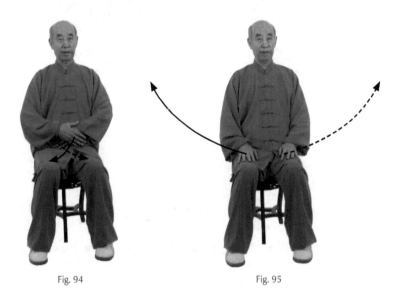

Fig. 94   Fig. 95

Step 1 Beginning of Heaven's Creation (*Qian Yuan Qi Yun*)

1. Guide to the movements

1) While breathing in, raise the anus, pull in the abdomen, and turn up the toes. At the same time, swing the palms to the right and left to shoulder level as the arms are rotated inward, palms facing backward, and arms naturally straight, eyes fixed on the left palm (Fig. 96). As the arms are turned outward, swing the palms facing down and level to in front of the body and shoulder-width apart, arms naturally straight, eyes fixed on both palms (Fig. 97).

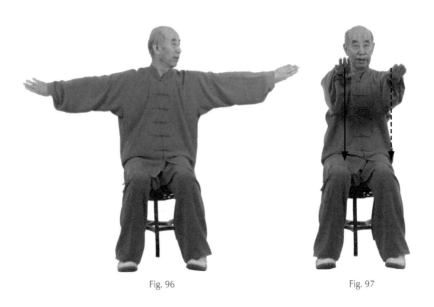

Fig. 96   Fig. 97

2) While breathing out, relax the abdomen and anus, toes grasping the ground. At the same time, drop both palms with the arms down to the *futu* acupoint, and sit with the body upright, eyes looking straight ahead (Fig. 98).

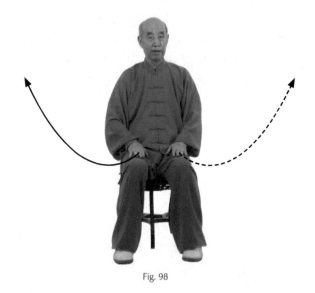

Fig. 98

3) While breathing in, raise the anus and pull in the abdomen, toes turned up. At the same time, turn the palms inward rotating from the elbows and swing them to shoulder level respectively to the left and right, palms facing backward, arms naturally straight, eyes fixed on the right palm (Fig. 99). Without stopping, turn the palms outward with the arms and swing them facing down and level to in front of the body, and shoulder-width apart. The arms should be naturally straight, eyes fixed on both palms (Fig. 100).

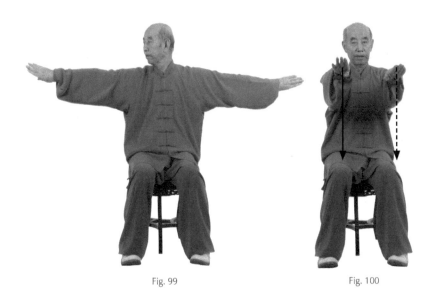

Fig. 99   Fig. 100

4) While breathing out, relax the abdomen and anus, toes grasping the ground. At the same time, drop both palms down to the *futu* acupoint, and sit with the body upright, eyes looking straight ahead (Fig. 101).

Do Movements 5, 6, 7 and 8 the same as Movements 1, 2, 3 and 4, but in the opposite direction.

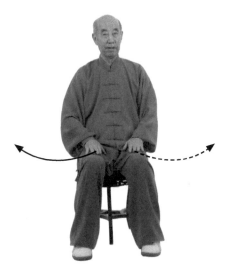

Fig. 101

3. *Number of times to practice*

Do one round.

4. Points for attention

1) Exert slight force with the thumbs to increase the range of rotations of the arms when rotating the arms inward and moving the palms apart.

2) Make the sound "*hu*" silently or concentrate the mind on *dantian*.

5. Main effects

1) It helps to smooth the hand-*taiyin* lung meridian and the hand-*yangming* large intestine meridian, and has a certain effect in preventing and treating diseases of the respiratory system, such as colds and bronchitis.

2) Concentration of the mind on the *dantian* helps to expel distracting thoughts, purify the cerebrum, invigorate the spleen, replenish *qi*, strengthen the body's resistance, consolidate the constitution and improve the physique.

3) Breathing in and turning the toes up to press the *yongquan* acupoint nourishes the kidneys, and breathing out and grasping the ground to stimulate the *yinbai* and *lidui* acupoints on the spleen and stomach meridians to nourish the spleen.

4) The traditional formula for respiration says: The exhaling sound of "*hu*" is attached to the spleen. Therefore, making the sound "*hu*" silently regulates the stomach function and invigorates the spleen.

Step 2 Double Fish Hung on the Wall (*Shuang Yu Xuan Ge*)

1. Guide to the movements

1) While breathing in, raise the anus, pull in the abdomen, turn up the toes, and turn the body about 45 degrees to the left. At the same time, rotate the palms with the arms inward, and swing them respectively to the left and right sides, palms about shoulder level, and palms facing backwards, eyes looking straight to the left (Fig. 102). While breathing out, relax the abdomen and anus, toes grasping the ground, and turn the body to the right. At the same time, rotate the left palm with the left arm outward, and move it back in front of the right lower abdomen, palm facing up, and move the right palm inward and drop it down on the left wrist, with the phalanx of the ring finger placed on the *taiyuan* acupoint as if feeling the pulse, eyes fixed on the hands (Fig. 103).

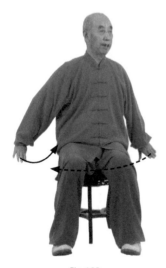

Fig. 102

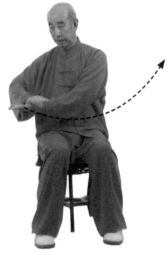

Fig. 103

2) While breathing in, raise the anus, pull in the abdomen, turn the toes up, and turn the body to the left. At the same time, keep the hands in the same posture as if feeling the pulse and swing them forward in curved lines to the left in front of the body, left arm naturally straight, and left palm facing up, eyes fixed on both palms (Fig. 104). While breathing out, relax the abdomen and anus, toes grasping the ground, and turn the body to the right to keep it upright. At the same time, rotate the left arm inward and the right arm outward. After twisting the finger on the *taiyuan* acupoint, place the right palm on the left in front of the chest, palm to palm and *laogong* acupoint to *laogong* acupoint. The palms should be about 20 cm from the chest, and the eyes should be fixed on both palms (Fig. 105).

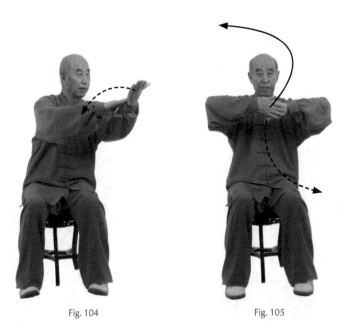

Fig. 104   Fig. 105

3) While breathing in, raise the anus, pull in the abdomen, and turn up the toes. At the same time, rub the palms to and fro horizontally, and then rotate the left palm with the left arm inward to press downward to the side of the left hip, about 20 cm from the hip, left arm bent in an arc, left fingers pointing to the right, and rotate the right palm with the right arm inward to raise the arm up above the head to the right, right arm bent in an arc, and right fingers pointing to the left, eyes looking straight to the left (Fig. 106).

4) While breathing out, relax the abdomen and anus, toes grasping the ground. At the same time, drop the right palm with the right arm to join the left palm and let them hang down by the sides of the body, eyes looking straight ahead (Fig. 107).

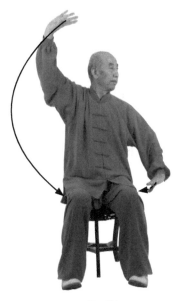

Fig. 106

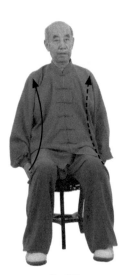

Fig. 107

Do Movements 5, 6, 7 and 8 the same as Movements 1, 2, 3 and 4, but in the opposite direction.

2. Number of times to practice

Do one round.

3. Points for attention

The same as those for the standing exercise.

4. Main effects

1) Helps to improve the function of the lungs and relieve disorders of the respiratory system such as cough and asthma.

2) Helps to improve the functions of the spleen and stomach, and relieve ailments of the digestive system such as indigestion and stomachache.

3) Helps to improve the function of the kidneys and has certain effect on the reproductive and urinary systems.

4) Breathing in and turning up the toes to press the *yongquan* acupoint nourishes the kidneys, and breathing out with the toes grasping the ground to stimulate the *yinbai* and *lidui* acupoints of the spleen and stomach meridians nourishes the spleen.

Step 3 Old Horse Stabled (*Lao Ji Fu Li*)

1. Guide to the movements

1) While breathing in, raise the anus, pull in the abdomen and turn up the toes. At the same time, rotate the palms with the arms outward, and swing them forward to shoulder level, palms facing up and shoulder-width apart, eyes fixed on both palms (Fig. 108). While breathing out, relax the abdomen and anus, toes grasping the ground. At the same time, clench the fists slowly and move them with the arms, elbows bent, back in front of the chest, elbows down, forearms touching each other against the body, fists at chin height, eyes looking straight ahead (Fig. 109).

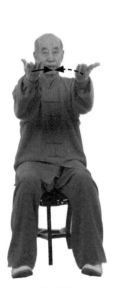

Fig. 108

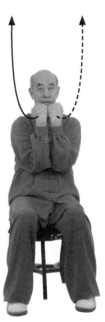

Fig. 109

2) While breathing in, raise the anus, pull in the abdomen and turn the toes up. At the same time, unclench the fists, rotate them inward and extend them forward and up, palms facing forward and shoulder-width apart, and arms naturally straight, eyes looking straight ahead (Fig. 110). While breathing out, relax the abdomen and anus, toes grasping the ground. At the same time, change the palms gradually into hooked hands (*shaoshang* and *shangyang* acupoints connected), and move them from the sides to hang behind the body, with the point of the hooks facing up, arms straight, eyes looking straight to the left (Fig. 111).

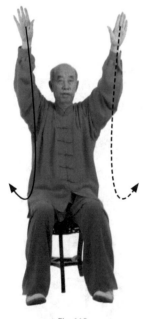

Fig. 110

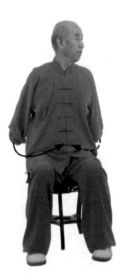

Fig. 111

3) While breathing in, raise the anus, pull in the abdomen, and turn the toes up. At the same time, change the hooked hands back into palms, and rotate them inward with the arms before the abdomen, the backs of the hands against each other, fingers facing down, eyes looking straight ahead (Fig. 112). Without stopping, raise the palms, with the backs against each other, bend the fingers one by one in order and then snap the fingernails before the face, and move them apart to the right and left sides of the body. Straighten them naturally, fingers facing up, wrists at shoulder level, eyes looking straight ahead (Figs. 113–115).

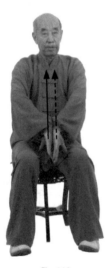

Fig. 112

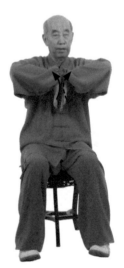
Fig. 113

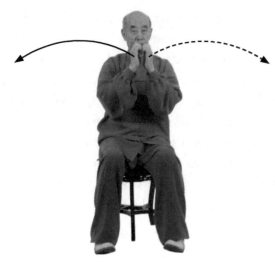

Fig. 114

4) While breathing out, relax the abdomen and anus, toes grasping the ground. At the same time, drop the palms downward slowly, and put them by the sides, eyes looking straight ahead (Fig. 116).

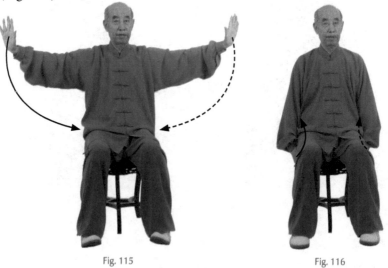

Fig. 115   Fig. 116

Do Movements 5, 6, 7 and 8 the same as Movements 1, 2, 3 and 4, but in the opposite direction.

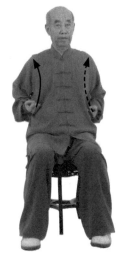

Fig. 117

2. *Number of times to practice*

Do one round. Clench the fists at the eighth movement, and place them by the waist to make preparations for Step 4 (Fig. 117).

3. *Points for attention*

1) It is appropriate to breathe in and breathe out once each at the first and second movements, and keep the breath deep, long and slow.

2) When clenching the fists with bent elbows in front of the chest, use the middle fingertip to touch the *laogong* acupoint.

3) Bend the wrists into hooked hands with a large range of movement.

4) Utter the sound "*dzer*" silently, and concentrate to direct the movements, or concentrate the mind on the *taiyuan* acupoint.

4. *Main effects*

1) Pressing the *laogong* acupoint helps to improve the function of the heart, and has a certain effect in relieving high blood pressure and coronary heart disease.

2) The movements of flexing the wrists into hooked hands, placing the wrists on top of each other and doubling the fingers helps to invigorate the heart and lungs as they have the effect of massaging *taiyuan*, the source acupoint of the lung meridian, *daling*, the source acupoint of the pericardium meridian, and *shenmen*, the source acupoint of the heart meridian.

3) Breathe in, and turn the toes up to press the *yongquan* acupoint to nourish the kidneys. Breathe out, grasping the ground with the toes to stimulate the *yinbai* and *lidui* acupoints of the spleen and stomach meridians to nourish the spleen.

4) Helps to nourish the spleen *qi* and increase the primordial *qi* to strengthen the body's resistance and improve the health.

Step 4 Ji Chang Shoots a Louse (*Ji Chang Guan Shi*)

1. Guide to the movements

1) While breathing in, raise the anus, pull in the abdomen, and turn the toes up. At the same time, unclench the fists and push the wrists forward, arms naturally straight, wrists about shoulder level, palms shoulder-width apart, and fingers facing up, eyes fixed on both palms (Fig. 118).

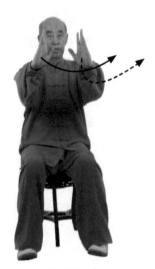

Fig. 118

2) While breathing out, relax the abdomen and anus, toes grasping the ground. At the same time, clench the fists loosely, move them horizontally to behind the body as the latter turns to the left, relax the left arm at shoulder level, bend the right arm, with the right elbow bent in front of the left side of the chest, eyes fixed on the left fist (Fig. 119). Without stopping, continue to turn the body to the left and hold that posture, left arm straight. Pull the right fist back to in front of the right side of the chest, clench the fists tightly, fingers touching the *laogong* acupoint, relax the chest and straighten the back, eyes fixed on the left fist (Fig. 120).

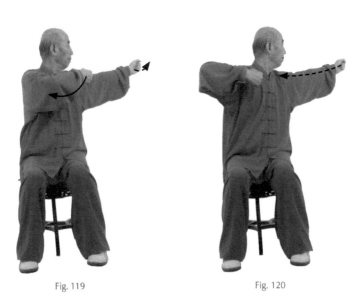

Fig. 119   Fig. 120

3) While breathing in, raise the anus, pull in the abdomen, and turn the toes up. At the same time, unclench the fists and rotate them inward with the arms. Move the arms horizontally to in front of the body, arms straight at shoulder level, palms facing down, eyes fixed on both palms (Fig. 121).

4) While breathing out, relax the abdomen and anus, toes grasping the ground. At the same time, drop the palms downward and clench the fists immediately, and move them back by the sides of the waist, palms facing up, eyes looking straight ahead (Fig. 122).

Do Movements 5, 6, 7 and 8 the same as Movements 1, 2, 3 and 4, but in the opposite direction.

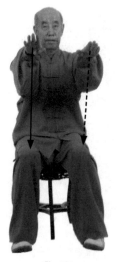

Fig. 121

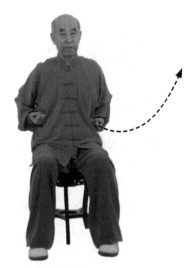

Fig. 122

2. Number of times to practice

Do two rounds.

3. Points for attention

1) When doing the movement of "pushing the palms forward" at the first movement it is appropriate for the force to originate at the root (shoulders), flow through the middle (elbows) and reach the tips (hands).

2) When doing the movement of "turning the body to the left" at the second movement it is appropriate to relax the neck, raise the head and keep the body upright.

3) When doing the third movement, it is appropriate to relax the whole body and swing both palms in front of the body.

4) When doing the fourth movement, raise the *baihui* acupoint, drop the shoulders and elbows with the hands down, and send *qi* to the *dantian*.

5) Concentrate the mind on the *mingmen* acupoint.

4. Main effects

1) Clenching the fists and touching the *laogong* acupoint help to clear the heart of heat and reduce the temperature.

2) Pulling the bow and shooting the arrow help to relax the chest, promote the normal flow of *qi*, and regulate the heart and lungs.

3) Concentrating the mind on the *mingmen* acupoint helps to nourish *yin* and the kidneys, and strengthen the kidneys and the waist.

Step 5 Bend the Body to Brush the Shoes (*Gong Shen Dan Xue*)
1. Guide to the movements

1) While breathing in, raise the anus, pull in the abdomen, turn the toes up, relax the chest, and expand the body and turn it to the left. At the same time, unclench the left fist, rotate the left arm inward and lift it up, eyes fixed on the left palm (Fig. 123). Without stopping, swing the left palm forward, above and to the right as the left arm is rotated outward and the body is turned to the right, left arm straight, eyes fixed on the left palm (Fig. 124). Without stopping, drop the left palm down to before the right shoulder (the back of the thumb and the radial side of the index finger against the

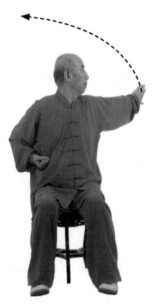

Fig. 123

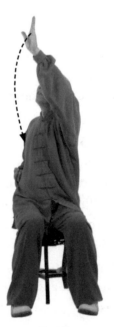

Fig. 124

right shoulder), bend the elbow and turn up the fingers, eyes fixed on the left palm (Fig. 125).

2) While breathing out, relax the abdomen and anus, toes grasping the ground, and bend the upper body forward to the right. At the same time, rotate the left palm outward slightly to rub from the right side of the waist downward to the thigh, shank and outer ankle (the phalanxes along the foot-*taiyang* bladder meridian, the palm along the foot-*shaoyang* gallbladder meridian and the palm base along the foot-*yangming* stomach meridian), head raised slightly (Fig. 126). Without stopping, turn the body to the left and keep it upright. At the same time, rotate the left palm inward with

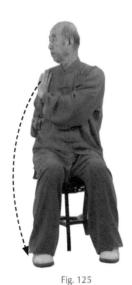

Fig. 125

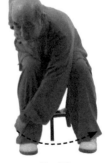

Fig. 126

the left arm to rub from the instep to the outer side of the left foot as if brushing the shoes, head raised slightly, eyes fixed on the left palm (Fig. 127).

3) While breathing in, raise the anus, pull in the abdomen, and turn the toes up. At the same time, rotate the left arm outward and clench the left fist, and raise it up to the left knee joint with a slight rise of the upper body, head slightly raised (Fig. 128).

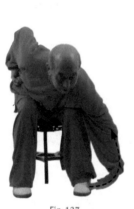
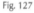

Fig. 127

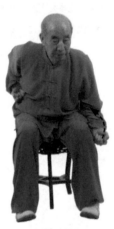

Fig. 128

4) While breathing out, relax the abdomen and anus, toes grasping the ground, with the upper part of the body rising. At the same time, move the left fist, fingers uppermost, back to the left side of the waist, the *zhongchong* acupoint at the tip of the middle finger touching the *laogong* acupoint at the center of the palm, eyes looking straight ahead (Fig. 129).

Do Movements 5, 6, 7 and 8 the same as Movements 1, 2, 3 and 4, but in the opposite direction.

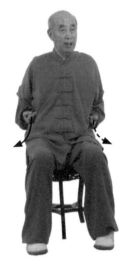

Fig. 129

2. Number of times to practice
Do two rounds.

3. Points for attention
1) Concentrate the mind on the *mingmen* acupoint.

2) Relax the body as much as possible, with a large range of movement. When bending forward as if to brush the shoes, beginners and people suffering from ailments should choose ranges of movement suitable for their abilities.

3) The body should be straightened slowly and at an even speed.

4. Main effects
The same as for the Standing Stance.

Step 6 Rhinoceros Gazes at the Moon (*Xi Niu Wang Yue*)

1. Guide to the movements

1) While breathing in, raise the anus, pull in the abdomen, and turn the toes up. At the same time, unclench the fists and rotate them with the arms inward. Press the palms down and back, palms facing down, eyes looking straight ahead (Fig. 130). Without stopping, let the hands hang loosely from the wrists, and press them downward, palms facing backward and fingers pointing down, eyes looking straight ahead (Fig. 131).

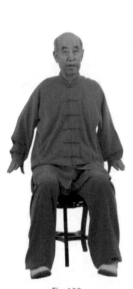

Fig. 130

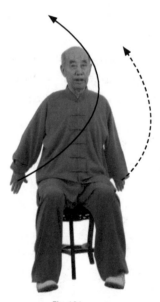

Fig. 131

2) While breathing out, relax the abdomen and anus, toes grasping the ground. At the same time, move the palms upward as the body is turned to the left, to snap the wrists and flash the palms forward above the head on the left and right sides, both arms curved, palms facing up and forward, fingers pointing to each other, eyes looking up and back to the left as if looking at the moon (Fig. 132).

3) While breathing in, raise the anus, pull in the abdomen, and turn the toes up. Turn the body to the right to keep it upright. At the same time, move the palms downward and swing them in a curved line to the front part of the chest as the arms are rotated outward, arms naturally straight, palms facing up and fingers facing forward, palms shoulder-width apart, eyes fixed on both palms (Fig. 133).

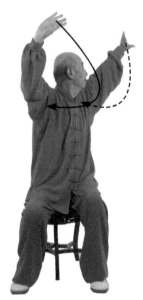
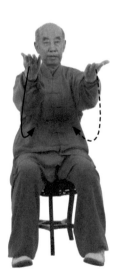

Fig. 132   Fig. 133

4) While breathing out, relax the abdomen and anus, toes grasping the ground. At the same time, after dropping the hands down by the sides of the body as the arms are rotated inward, clench the fists and move them back to the sides of the waist, fingers facing up, eyes looking straight ahead (Fig. 134).

Do Movements 5, 6, 7 and 8 the same as Movements 1, 2, 3 and 4, but in the opposite direction.

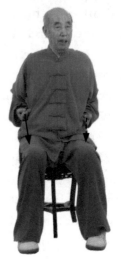

Fig. 134

2. Number of times to practice

Do two rounds, and drop the palms on the *futu* acupoint in the upright sitting position, eyes looking straight ahead (Fig. 135).

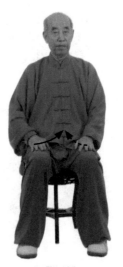

Fig. 135

3. Points for attention

1) Concentrate the mind on the *mingmen* acupoint.

2) It is appropriate to keep the body upright with a big range of movement, but it varies from person to person, and for old and weak people, and lumbago sufferers.

3) When clenching the fists, the *zhongchong* meridian acupoint touches the *laogong* acupoint momentarily.

4) Rotate the arms with a big range of movement at an even speed. Be sure not to stiffen the shoulders.

4. Main effects

The same as for the Standing Stance.

Step 7 Lotus Flower Appears Above the Water (*Fu Rong Chu Shui*)

1. Guide to the movements

1) While breathing in, raise the anus, pull in the abdomen, and turn up the toes. At the same time, keep the backs of the hands against each other in front of the abdomen, fingers facing down, eyes looking straight ahead (Fig. 136). Without stopping, place the backs of the palms against each other, bend the carpuses, the metacarpal bones, the first phalanxes, the second phalanxes and the third phalanxes of the fingers one by one in order, and then snap the fingernails, unclench the fists, and move them apart to the two sides, palms facing up and as high as shoulder level, and arms naturally straight, eyes looking straight ahead (Figs. 137–139).

Movements

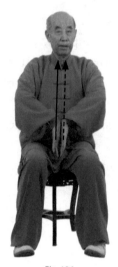

Fig. 136

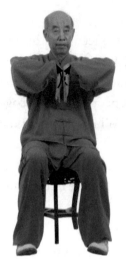

Fig. 137

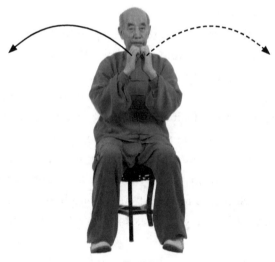

Fig. 138

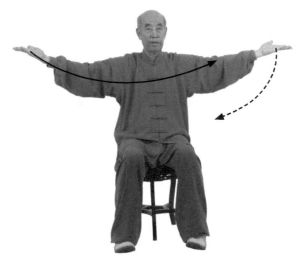

Fig. 139

2) While breathing out, relax the abdomen and anus, toes grasping the ground. At the same time, clench the left fist as the body turns to the left and the left arm is rotated inward, and drop it slightly, fingers facing down. Clench the right fist as the right arm is rotated inward, and proceed to swing it forward horizontally to the left, fingers facing down, eyes fixed on the right fist (Fig. 140).

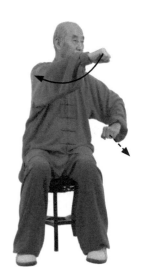

Fig. 140

Without stopping, turn the body to the right to keep it upright. At the same time, drop the left fist down by the left hip, left arm bent in a curve, and turn the wrist up, thumb side facing back, fist about 30 cm from the hip; move the right fist back to in front of the right side of the chest as the right arm is rotated inward, thumb part facing down, fist about 30 cm from the chest, eyes looking straight to the left (Fig. 141).

3) While breathing in, raise the anus, pull in the abdomen, and turn the toes up. At the same time, unclench the fists, drop the right arm down, the wrists against each other, and hold the hands up in front of the chest in the posture of a blooming lotus flower, eyes fixed on both palms (Fig. 142). Without stopping, hold the

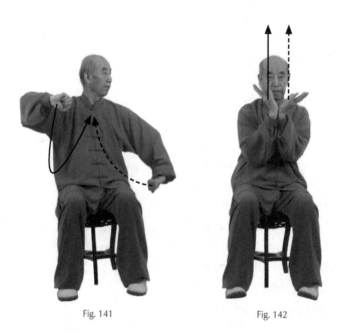

Fig. 141   Fig. 142

palms still further up in the posture of a blooming lotus flower, arms naturally straight, eyes fixed on both palms (Fig. 143).

4) While breathing out, relax the abdomen and anus, toes grasping the ground. At the same time, drop the palms down by the two sides of the body, eyes looking straight ahead (Fig. 144).

Do Movements 5, 6, 7 and 8 the same as Movements 1, 2, 3 and 4, but in the opposite direction.

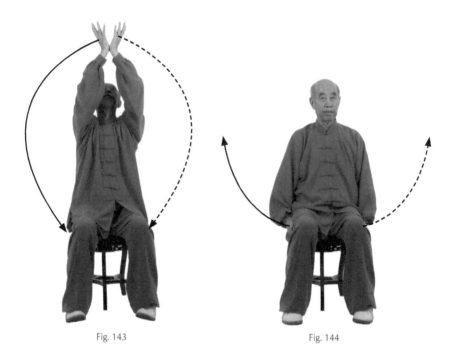

Fig. 143   Fig. 144

2. Number of times to practice

Do one round.

3. Points for attention

1) When bending the fingers and snapping the fingernails at the first movement, the movements of the shoulders, elbows, wrists and fingers should be continuous. Do the movements in an easy and elegant manner.

2) At the second movement, one arm is bent by the hip and the other moved back to in front of the chest. The movements must be coordinated, with equal attention given to the hands and feet. It should look just like a lotus flower floating on top of the water.

3) At the third movement, hold up the palms, the wrists touching, in the symbolic form of a lotus flower appearing above the water in a clear pond and in a soothing breeze. Its lofty moral quality of "coming up from the mud without being contaminated by it" will give people the feeling of its cleanness and honesty.

4) At the fourth movement, raise the *baihui* acupoint at the top of the head, drop the shoulders, straighten the neck, and drop the elbows for the hands to hang by the sides.

5) Utter the sound *"dzer"* silently or concentrate the mind on the *taiyuan* acupoint.

4. Main effects

1) Removal of obstacles from the three *yin* and three *yang* meridians of the hand helps to strengthen the heart, nourish the lungs, moisten the intestines, resolve the nodes and regulate the *Sanjiao* meridian.

2) Removal of obstacles from the three *yin* and three *yang* meridians of the foot helps to regulate the stomach, invigorate the spleen, soothe the liver, promote the function of the gallbladder, and strengthen the kidneys and waist.

3) This step with the waist as the axis to drive the upper limbs acts on the *Du* and bladder meridians, and helps to nourish *yin* and the kidneys, and strengthen the muscles and bones.

Step 8 Golden Rooster Heralds the Dawn (*Jin Ji Bao Xiao*)

1. Guide to the movements

1) While breathing in, raise the anus, pull in the abdomen, heels up, and raise the *baihui* acupoint at the top of the head. At the same time, change the palms gradually into hooked hands, and swing them upward respectively to the two sides, arms naturally straight, and wrists about shoulder level, eyes fixed on the left hooked hand (Fig. 145).

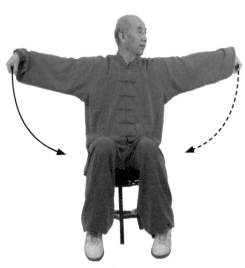

Fig. 145

2) While breathing out, relax the abdomen and anus, heels on the ground. At the same time, change the hooked hands into palms, and press them down by the sides with the elbows dropped in a curved line, arms naturally straight, palms facing down and fingers outward, eyes looking straight ahead (Fig. 146).

3) While breathing in, raise the anus, pull in the abdomen, and bend and raise the left leg, toes facing down. At the same time, while rotating the arms inward, move the palms before the abdomen and change them into hooked hands. Then extend them forward and upward to the left and right sides of the head forward and above, arms straight and hook tips facing down, eyes looking straight ahead (Fig. 147).

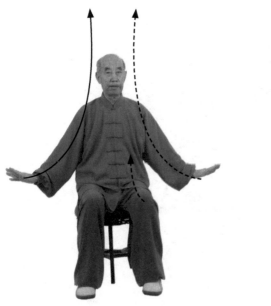

Fig. 146

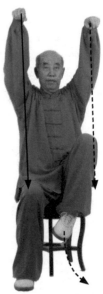

Fig. 147

4) While breathing out, relax the abdomen and anus, drop the left foot and return it to the original position. At the same time, change the hooked hands into palms and press them on the *futu* acupoint, eyes looking straight ahead (Fig. 148).

Do Movements 5, 6, 7 and 8 the same as Movements 1, 2, 3 and 4, but in the opposite direction.

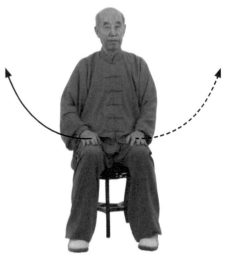

Fig. 148

2. Number of times to practice

Do one round.

3. Points for attention

1) Concentrate the mind on the *dantian* (referring to the *guanyuan* acupoint here).

2) Keep the upper and lower limbs coordinated, relaxed and soft, natural and elegant. Raise the *baihui* acupoint, and look into the distance.

3) While swinging the hooked hands to the sides and extending the bent wrists upward relax the chest, straighten the body and neck, and keep the head erect.

4. Main effects

1) Pulling the heels up to press the *yongquan* acupoint helps to stimulate the foot-*shaoyin* kidney meridian to nourish *yin* and the kidneys.

2) Swinging the hooked hands helps to remove obstacles from the source acupoints of the three *yin* and three *yang* of the hand meridians, removing obstruction from the meridians and collaterals, nourishing the heart and lungs, regulating *Sanjiao* meridian, moistening the intestines and resolving the nodes.

Step 9 Wild Geese Land on the Beach (*Ping Sha Luo Yan*)

1. Guide to the movements

1) While breathing in, raise the anus, and pull in the abdomen, heels up. At the same time, swing the arms with the hands hanging down from the wrists respectively to both sides of the body in a curved line to shoulder level, eyes fixed on the right palm

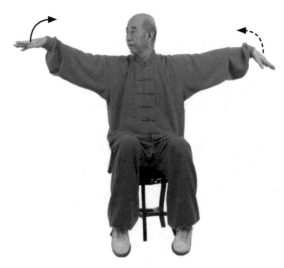

Fig. 149

(Fig. 149). Without stopping, lower the elbows, and draw the hands back in an arc, palms at shoulder level and facing down, eyes fixed on the right palm (Fig. 150).

2) While breathing out, relax the abdomen and anus, heels on the ground. At the same time, move the arms with the elbows straight and the hands hanging from the wrists, and push them in curved lines to the sides, both arms naturally straight, wrists at shoulder level, palms facing outward and fingers facing up, eyes fixed on the right palm (Fig. 151).

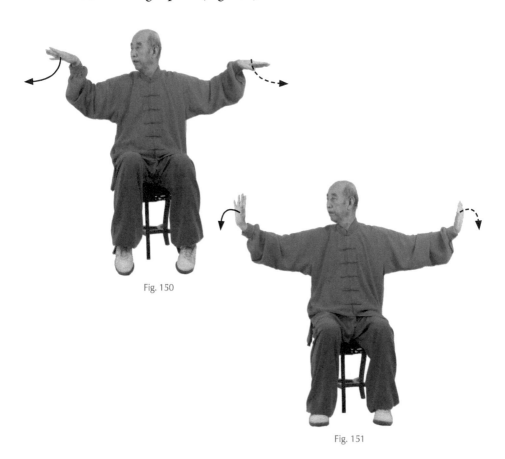

Fig. 150

Fig. 151

3) While breathing in, raise the anus and pull in the abdomen, heels up. At the same time, extend the palms to the two sides, palms facing down and arms naturally straight. Then, move the palms downward with the arms, elbows bent, and draw them back in an arc form, palms as high as shoulder level, palms facing down, eyes fixed on the right palm (Fig. 152).

4) The same as Movement 2 (Fig. 153).

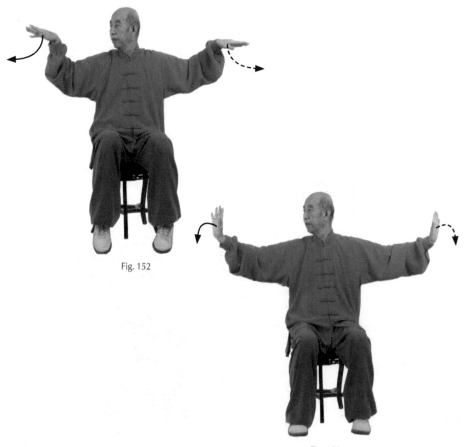

Fig. 152

Fig. 153

5) While breathing in, raise the anus and pull in the abdomen, heels up. At the same time, extend the hands slightly to the sides and move them upward, arms naturally straight, palms facing down, eyes fixed on the right palm (Fig. 154).

6) While breathing out, relax the abdomen and anus, heels on the ground. At the same time, drop the elbows to the sides, fingers facing down, eyes looking straight ahead (Fig. 155). Alternate the directions of the movements.

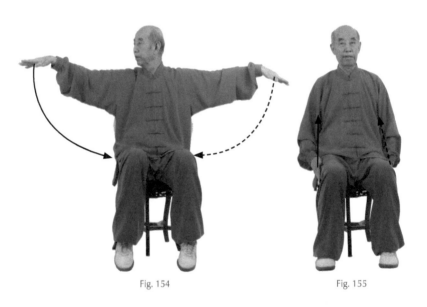

Fig. 154   Fig. 155

2. Number of times to practice

Six repetitions in each direction.

3. Points for attention

1) Concentrate the mind on the *laogong* acupoint.

2) Keep the upper and lower limbs coordinated. Relax the chest and straighten the back when breathing in, and pull the chest slightly in and relax the waist when breathing out.

3) When pushing the palms to the sides, the force should originate at the root (shoulders), flow through the middle (elbows) and reach the tips (hands). When both hands are lowered, the shoulders and elbows should be lowered at the same time.

4. Main effects

1) Concentrating the mind on the *laogong* acupoint helps to regulate the hand-*jueyin* pericardium meridian, relieving the heart and regulating the flow of the blood.

2) Raising and lowering the heels helps to remove obstructions from the meridians of the three *yin* and three *yang* of the foot, and has a certain effect in improving the functions of the spleen, stomach, liver, gallbladder and kidneys.

Step 10 White Crane Flies High in the Clouds
(*Yun Duan Bai He*)

1. Guide to the movements

1) While breathing in, raise the anus and pull in the abdomen, toes turned up. At the same time, move the *hegu* acupoints on the hands and rub them upward as the arms are rotated inward to near the *dabao* acupoint on the lateral side of the chest and on the middle auxiliary line in the 6th intercostal space, eyes looking straight ahead (Fig. 156). Without stopping, rotate the palms with

the *hegu* acupoints as the axis as the arms are rotated outward, so that the fingers face back, eyes looking straight ahead (Fig. 157).

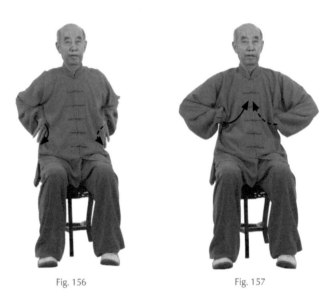

Fig. 156   Fig. 157

2) While breathing out, relax the abdomen and anus, toes grasping the ground. At the same time, press the backs of the hands against the *dabao* acupoint, and then put one on top of the other in front of the chest, both arms bent, fingers facing inward, eyes looking straight ahead (Fig. 158). Without stopping, rotate the hands, palms up and with the fingers bent, and swing them respectively to the left and right, arms naturally straight and at shoulder level, and palms facing forward, eyes looking straight ahead (Fig. 159).

Movements

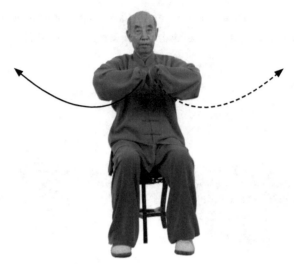

Fig. 158

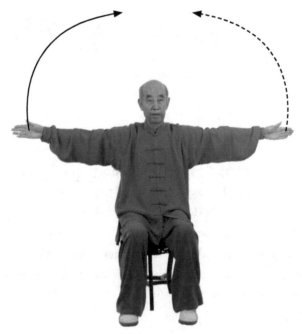

Fig. 159

3) While breathing in, raise the anus and pull in the abdomen, toes turned up. At the same time, swing the palms up and forward above the head on both sides as the arms are rotated inward, to snap the wrists and flash the palms, both arms bent in an arc form, eyes looking straight ahead (Fig. 160).

4) While breathing out, relax the abdomen and anus, toes grasping the ground. At the same time, drop the hands down the respective sides, palms facing inward, eyes looking straight ahead (Fig. 161).

Do Movements 5, 6, 7 and 8 the same as Movements 1, 2, 3 and 4.

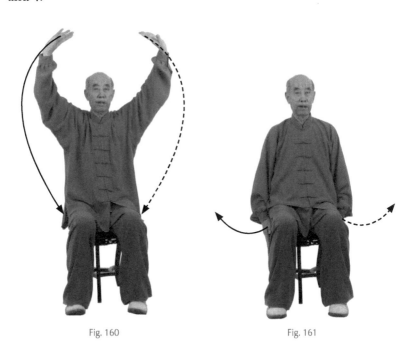

Fig. 160   Fig. 161

2. Number of times to practice

Do one round.

3. Points for attention

1) At the first movement, relax the chest, straighten the back, and keep the head erect while breathing in and turning up the toes.

2) At the second movement, swing the palms after the fingers are doubled one by one in order to ensure that the "four folds" are continuous.

3) At the third movement, swing the hands upward, dangling from the wrists, then snap the wrists and flash the palms, keeping the ends of the middle fingers and the *jianyu* acupoint on the shoulders basically at the same level.

4) At the fourth movement, raise the *baihui* acupoint, and drop the shoulders and elbows together with the hands, with the *qi* flowing to the *dantian*.

5) Concentrate the mind on the *dantian* (referring to the *guanyuan* acupoint).

4. Main effects

The same as for the Standing Stance.

Step 11 Phoenix Salutes the People (*Feng Huang Lai Yi*)

1. Guide to the movements

1) While breathing in, raise the anus, pull in the abdomen, and turn the body about 30º to the left. At the same time, swing the palms as the arms are rotated inward to behind the body, eyes looking straight ahead (Fig. 162). Then swing the palms forward as the arms are rotated outward from the sides to shoulder level on either side, arms naturally straight and palms shoulder-width apart and facing up, eyes looking straight ahead to the left (Fig. 163).

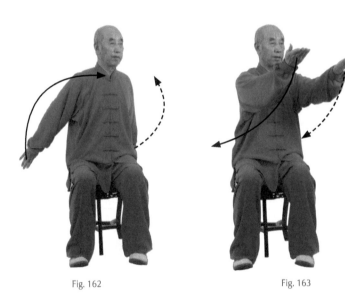

Fig. 162   Fig. 163

2) While breathing out, relax the abdomen and anus, toes grasping the ground. At the same time, rotate the arms inward and change the palms gradually into hooked hands (*shaoshang* and *shangyang* acupoints connected), which are then stretched behind the body, arms naturally straight and hook tips facing up, eyes looking straight ahead to the left (Fig. 164).

3) While breathing in, raise the anus, pull in the abdomen, turn the toes up, and turn the body to the right to keep it upright. At the same time, change the hooked hands into palms, move them from the sides of the waist and cross them in front of the chest, left palm inside and both palms facing inward, eyes fixed on both palms (Fig. 165).

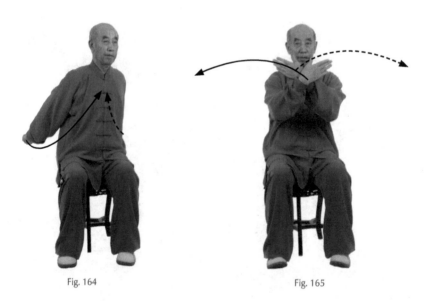

Fig. 164   Fig. 165

Without stopping, rotate the arms, move them apart before the face on either side, arms naturally straight, wrists about shoulder level and fingers facing up, eyes looking straight ahead (Fig. 166).

4) While breathing out, relax the abdomen and anus, toes grasping the ground. Move the left foot next to the right foot to keep them together, and straighten the bent legs. At the same time, drop the arms down the sides, palms facing inward, eyes looking straight ahead (Fig. 167).

Do Movements 5, 6, 7 and 8 the same as Movements 1, 2, 3 and 4, but in the opposite direction.

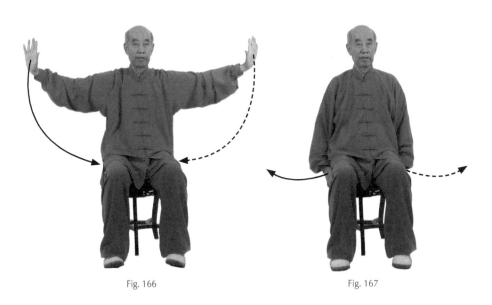

Fig. 166   Fig. 167

2. Number of times to practice

Do one round.

3. Points for attention

1) At the first movement, raise the *baihui* acupoint at the top of the head, keep the body upright and turn the spinal column to drive the arms apart and make them swing forward.

2) At the second movement, straighten the neck and raise the head, swing the palms back, bend the wrists to form hooked hands after the fingers are doubled one by one in order, and exert force slightly for a short moment.

3) At the third movement, when moving the hands apart in front of the chest and facing left and right alternately, keep the chest relaxed and the back straight, and drop the shoulders and elbows.

4) At the fourth movement, relax the whole body and drop the elbows and hands.

5) Concentrate the mind on the *dantian* and utter the sound "*hu*" softly.

4. Main effects

The same as for the Standing Stance.

Step 12 *Qi* and Breath Return to the Origin (*Qi Xi Gui Yuan*)

1. Guide to the movements

1) While breathing in, raise the anus, pull in the abdomen and turn the toes up. At the same time, rotate the arms first inward and then outward, and swing them respectively to the two sides of the body, palms changing from facing backward to facing forward. The angle between the arms and the upper body should be about 60 degrees, arms naturally straight, eyes looking straight ahead (Figs. 168 and 169).

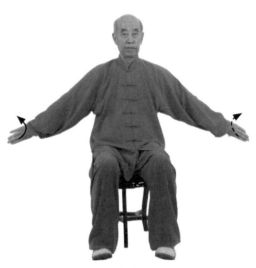

Fig. 168

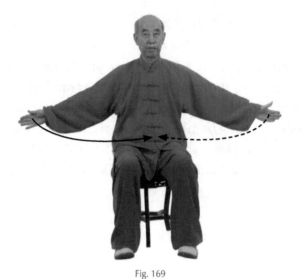

Fig. 169

2) While breathing out, relax the abdomen and anus, toes grasping the ground. At the same time, move the palms back and inward to form a circle before the lower abdomen, and return the *qi* of essence from the sun and the moon to the *guanyuan* acupoint, eyes looking straight ahead (Fig. 170).

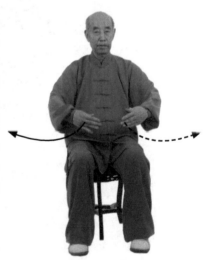

Fig. 170

3) While breathing in, raise the anus, pull in the abdomen and turn up the toes. At the same time, rotate the palms with the arms first inward and then outward, and swing them respectively to the two sides of the body, palms changing from facing backward to facing forward. The angle between the arms and the upper body should be about 60 degrees, arms naturally straight, eyes looking straight ahead (Figs. 171 and 172).

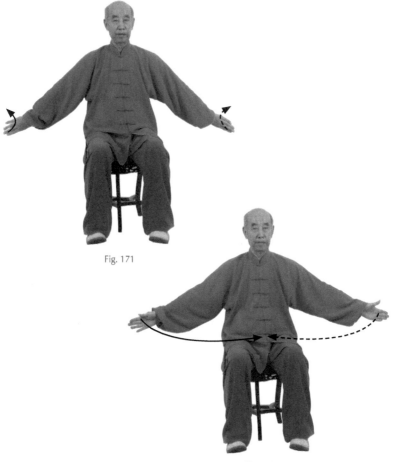

Fig. 171

Fig. 172

4) The same as Movement 2.

5) The same as Movement 3.

6) The same as Movement 2.

2. Number of times to practice

Do three rounds, breathing in once and breathing out once at each round.

3. Points for attention

1) Concentrate the mind on the collection of *qi* for the *guanyuan* acupoint.

2) When breathing in, raise the *baihui* acupoint at the top of the head, and when breathing out, relax the waist slightly, chest in.

3) When moving the palms back and inward to collect *qi* of essence from the sun and the moon, pay attention to narrowing the passage for the flow of *qi* to accelerate its flow.

4. Main effects

The *guanyuan* acupoint is located on the *Ren* meridian, and is one of the acupoints of the *dantian*. It is the meeting point for the three *yin* meridian of the foot and the *Ren* meridian, and one of the front *mu* points of the small intestine meridian. TCM calls it the "major acupoint of long life," and it has a noticeable effect in preserving health. Therefore, using the mind to draw *qi* for the *guanyuan* acupoint helps to invigorate the *qi* of the central *qi*, nourish the original *qi*, nourish the internal organs, and regulate *yin* and *yang*.

Ending Stance

1. Guide to the movements

1) While breathing in, raise the anus, pull in the abdomen, and turn the toes up. At the same time, rotate the palms with the arms first inward and then outward, and swing them respectively to the sides of the body, change the direction of the palms from facing backward to facing forward, the included angle between the arms and the upper body being about 60 degrees, arms naturally straight, eyes looking straight ahead (Figs. 173 and 174)

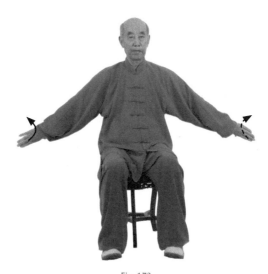

Fig. 173

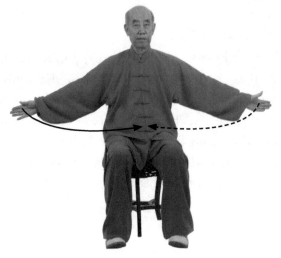

Fig. 174

2) While breathing out,
relax the abdomen and anus,
toes grasping the ground. At
the same time, move the palms
back and inward to form a
circle, and put one on top of
the other, facing inward, at the
guanyuan acupoint, left hand
inside for the male and right
hand inside for the female, eyes
lightly closed (Fig. 175).

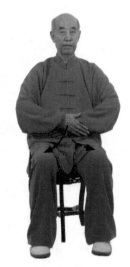

Fig. 175

3) Execute the movement of the "red dragon (tongue) stirs the sea," three times each to the left and right sides of the mouth so as to increase the elixir (saliva) and swallow it in three gulps.

4) Drop the palms down onto the *futu* acupoints, feet together, and close the exercise slowly to finish the whole practice session (Figs. 176 and 177)

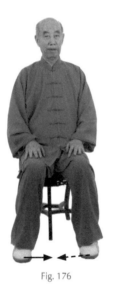 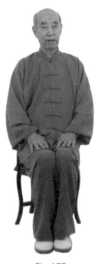

Fig. 176   Fig. 177

2. Points for attention

The same as for the Standing Stance.

3. Main effects

The same as for the Standing Stance.

Acupuncture Points

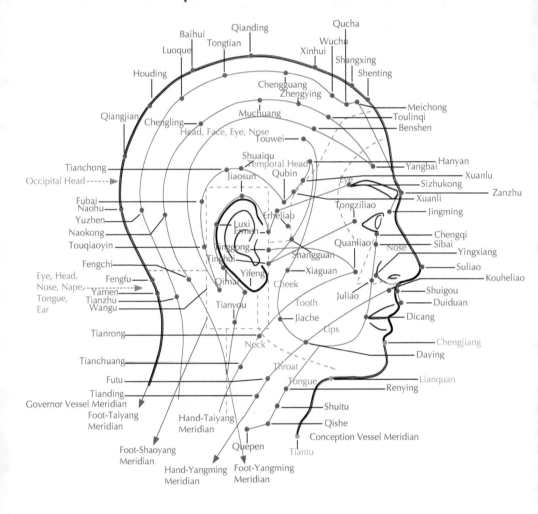

Acupoints on the head and face

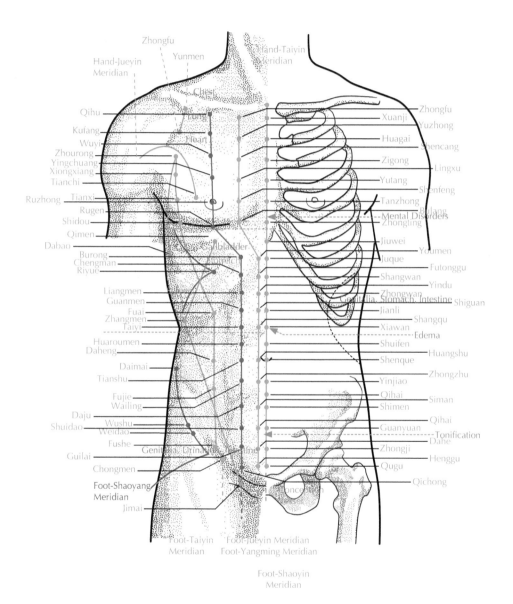

Acupoints on the chest and abdomen

139

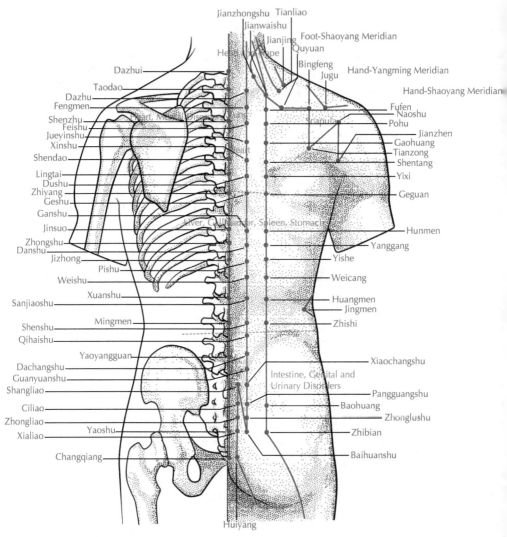

Governor Vessel Foot-Taiyang Meridian

Jianzhongshu Tianliao
Jianwaishu
Jianjing
Hua... pe Quyuan
Foot-Shaoyang Meridian
Dazhui
Bingfeng
Jugu Hand-Yangming Meridian
Taodao
Hand-Shaoyang Meridian
Dazhu
Fengmen
Shenzhu Fufen
Feishu Naoshu
Jueyinshu Pohu
Xinshu Scapula
Jianzhen
Shendao Gaohuang
Tianzong
Lingtai Shentang
Dushu
Zhiyang Yixi
Geshu
Ganshu Geguan
Jinsuo
Zhongshu Hunmen
Danshu
Jizhong Yanggang
Pishu Yishe
Weishu Weicang
Xuanshu
Sanjiaoshu Huangmen
Mingmen Jingmen
Shenshu Zhishi
Qihaishu
Yaoyangguan
Dachangshu Xiaochangshu
Guanyuanshu
Shangliao Pangguangshu
Ciliao Baohuang
Zhongliao Zhonglushu
Xialiao Yaoshu Zhibian
Changqiang Baihuanshu

Huiyang

Foot-Taiyang Meridian

Acupoints on the back and lumbar region

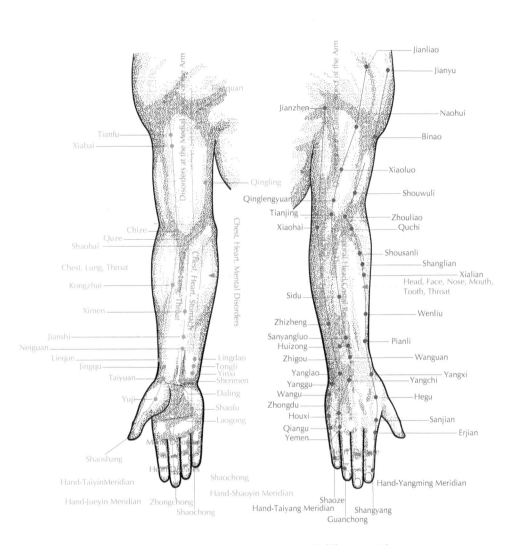

Acupoints in the upper limbs

141

Appendix
Acupuncture Points

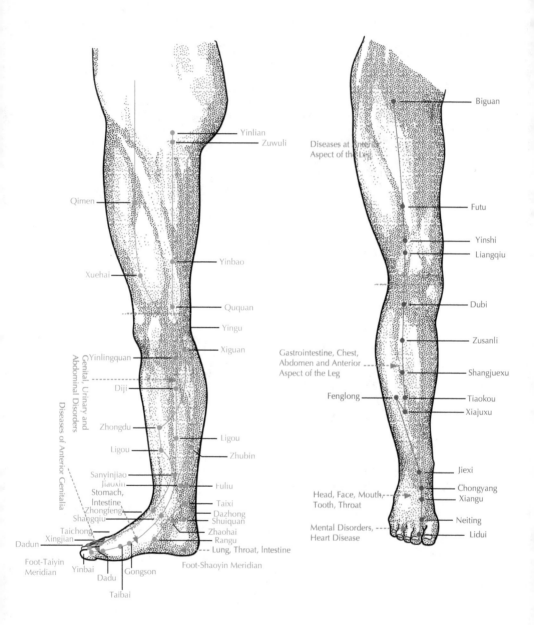

Acupoints in the lower limbs

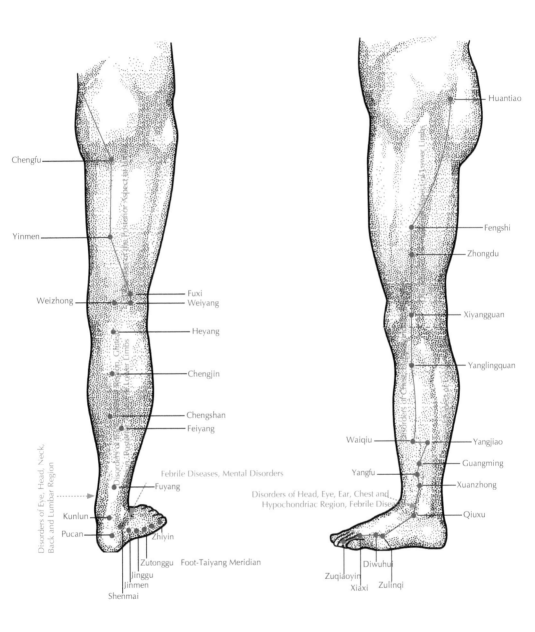

Chengfu

Yinmen

Weizhong

Fuxi
Weiyang

Heyang

Chengjin

Chengshan
Feiyang

Febrile Diseases, Mental Disorders

Fuyang

Disorders of Eye, Head, Neck,
Back and Lumbar Region

Kunlun

Pucan

Zhiyin

Zutonggu

Jinggu
Jinmen

Shenmai

Foot-Taiyang Meridian

Huantiao

Fengshi

Zhongdu

Xiyangguan

Yanglingquan

Waiqiu

Yangjiao

Guangming

Yangfu

Xuanzhong

Disorders of Head, Eye, Ear, Chest and
Hypochondriac Region, Febrile Dise

Qiuxu

Zuqiaoyin

Diwuhui

Xiaxi

Zulinqi

Acupoints in the lower limbs

143